Navigating
Smell and Taste
Disorders

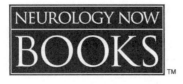

NEUROLOGY NOW
BOOKS
™

Lisa M. Shulman, MD
Series Editor-in-Chief
Fellow of the American Academy of Neurology

Professor of Neurology and Co-Director
of the University of Maryland Parkinson's Disease
and Movement Disorders Center

The Eugenia Brin Professor in Parkinson's Disease and
Movement Disorders

The Rosalyn Newman Distinguished Scholar
in Parkinson's Disease
University of Maryland School of Medicine
BALTIMORE, MARYLAND

Navigating
Smell and Taste
Disorders

Ronald DeVere, MD
Fellow of American Academy of Neurology
Fellow of American Academy of Disability
Evaluating Physicians
Director
Taste and Smell Disorders Clinic
AUSTIN, TEXAS

Marjorie Calvert
Catering Manager and Food Consultant
Taste and Smell Disorders Clinic
AUSTIN, TEXAS

demos
HEALTH
New York

Acquisitions Editor: Noreen Henson
Cover Design: Anthony Kosner, Wing & Ko.
Interior Page Design: Judy Gilats
Compositor: Publication Services, Inc.
Printer: Hamilton Printing Company

Visit our web site at www.demosmedpub.com.

Medical information provided by Demos Health, in the absence of a visit with a healthcare professional, must be considered as an educational service only. This book is not designed to replace a physician's independent judgment about the appropriateness or risks of a procedure or therapy for a given patient. Our purpose is to provide you with information that will help you make your own healthcare decisions.

The information and opinions provided here are believed to be accurate and sound, based on the best judgment available to the authors, editors, and publisher, but readers who fail to consult appropriate health authorities assume the risk of any injuries. The publisher and the author are not responsible for errors or omissions. The editors and publisher welcome any reader to report to the publisher any discrepancies or inaccuracies noticed.

The authors do not intend for this information to serve as a substitute for medical advice; any health concerns should be under supervision of a doctor. In addition, every effort was made to check the gluten-free status of the foods listed, however manufacturers are often changing formulas, so always double check the gluten-free status of your foods.

Disclosure statements provided by the authors are available upon request from the American Academy of Neurology, 1080 Montreal Avenue, St. Paul, MN 55110; Attn: Neurology Now Books.

Library of Congress Cataloging-in-Publication Data

DeVere, Ronald.
    Navigating smell and taste disorders / Ronald DeVere, Marjorie Calvert
        p. ; cm.
    Includes bibliographical references and index.
    ISBN 978-1-932603-96-5
    1. Smell disorders.   2. Taste disorders.   I. Calvert, Marjorie.
    [DNLM: 1. Olfaction Disorders.   2. Taste Disorders. WV 301 D491n 2011]
    RF341.D48 2011
    616.8'56—dc22

                                                                    2010013655

Special discounts on bulk quantities of Demos Health books are available to corporations, professional associations, pharmaceutical companies, health care organizations, and other qualifying groups. For details, please contact:

Special Sales Department
Demos Medical Publishing
11 W. 42nd Street, 15th Floor
New York, NY 10036
Phone: 800–532–8663 or 212–683–0072
Fax: 212–941–7842
E-mail: rsantana@demosmedpub.com

Made in the United States of America
  11 12 13   5 4 3 2

Contents

Foreword by Richard L. Doty, PhD   ix

Preface   xi

About the AAN Neurology Now Books Series
by Lisa M. Shulman, MD   xiii

Acknowledgments   xvii

Introduction   xix

CHAPTER 1
Why Can't I Smell?   1
Common Causes of Smell Disorders   1

CHAPTER 2
Why Can't I Taste?   21
Common Causes of Taste Disorders   22

CHAPTER 3
Temperature, Texture, and Spice:
How Does the Smell and Taste System Work?   33
How We Smell   33
How We Remember Odors   37
How We Taste   38

CHAPTER 4
Sniffing Out What's Wrong: How Smell and
Taste Disorders Are Diagnosed   49
Which Doctor to See? Seeking Medical Help   49
Visiting a Smell and Taste Clinic   52
Specialized Smell Testing   53
Specialized Taste Testing   56

CHAPTER 5

What Does It Mean? Treatment Options and Lifestyle Changes   61

Education about Your Disorder   62
Treatment for Smell and Taste Disorders   62
Living Well with a Smell and Taste Disorder   72
Potential New Treatments   77
Looking to the Future   78

CHAPTER 6

Food Preparation   81

General Information   81
Five Basic Tastes, Unlimited Flavors   86
Food Preparation Methods Suggested by Patients with
    Smell and Taste Disorders   88

Recipes   89

Introduction   90
Salads   93
Sides   99
Snacks and Appetizers   105
Fish and Seafood   109
Chicken   115
Beef   119
Condiments   127
Marinades and Sauces   135
Tips for Holiday Meals   147
Recipe Credits   151

Appendix A: Smell and Taste Clinics   153

Appendix B: Food Resources   157

Appendix C: Recommended Reading   159

Appendix D: Internet Resources   161

Appendix E: About Neurologists   163

Appendix F: About the American Academy of Neurology and
          the American Academy of Neurology Foundation   165

Glossary   167
Index   173

Foreword

Loss or distortion of the senses of smell and taste are very debilitating. Many patients with such problems suffer needlessly, and are commonly spurned by the medical community and come to believe they have anomalies for which nothing is known.

Navigating Smell and Taste Disorders is an informative overview of the nature of smell and taste disturbances and of the assessment and treatment options that are currently available. Melding the expertise of a neurologist with that of a food consultant, this unique and readable volume will be an invaluable resource for those afflicted with chemosensory dysfunction, as well as for spouses, caregivers, nurses, nutritionists, psychologists, and physicians who care for persons with such dysfunction.

This modest volume succinctly summarizes available information in a practical way with an emphasis on improving quality of life. Most notably, Dr. DeVere and Ms. Calvert outline a number of unique approaches to cooking to enhance the flavor sensations in patients with lessened smell and taste function, including a number of recipes that will aid in the enjoyment of life.

Richard L. Doty, PhD

Director
Smell and Taste Center

Professor
Department of Otorhinolaryngology
Head and Neck Surgery
University of Pennsylvania

PHILADELPHIA, PENNSYLVANIA

Preface

The idea for this book came about because our patients and their caregivers needed a concise source of information about smell and taste, and, specifically, disorders of smell and taste. We started looking in bookstores and on the Internet for books on this topic and found several medical and scientific books. However, they were totally unsuitable for the public, both in content and terminology. Therefore, I decided to write a handbook that offers basic knowledge, practical hints, and case examples for those dealing with these disorders. We believe this book will also be of value for health care providers such as nurse practitioners; physician assistants; family practitioners; geriatricians; internists; neurologists; and ear, nose, and throat physicians.

The book covers the smell, taste, and sensory (trigeminal) systems, and how they work individually and together to enable you to enjoy your food and appreciate everyday aromas. It also discusses the disorders of smell and taste and their effect on your daily life. It offers a practical guide to food preparation and sample recipes, which we think you will find to be among the most helpful parts of the book.

Ronald DeVere, MD

Marjorie Calvert

About the AAN Neurology Now Books™ Series

Here is a question for you: If you know more about your neurologic condition, will you do better than if you know less?

Well, it's not simply optimism—hard data shows that individuals who are more knowledgeable about their medical condition *do have better outcomes.* So, learning about your neurologic condition plays an important role in doing the very best you can. The main purpose of both the American Academy of Neurology's Neurology Now Books series and *Neurology Now®* magazine is to focus on the needs of people with neurologic disorders. Our goal is to view neurologic issues through the eyes of people with neurologic problems in order to understand and respond to their practical day-to-day needs.

So you are probably saying, *"Of course, knowledge is a good thing, but how can it change the course of my disease?"* Well, health care is really a two-way street. You need to find a knowledgeable and trusted neurologist; however, no physician can overcome the obstacle of working with inaccurate or incomplete information. Your physician is working to navigate the clues you provide in your own words, combined with the clues from their neurologic examination, in order to arrive at an accurate diagnosis and respond to your individual needs. Many types of important clues exist, such as your description of your symptoms or your ability to identify how your neurologic condition affects your daily activities. Poor patient-physician communication inevitably results in less-than-ideal outcomes. This problem is well-described by the old adage, "garbage in, garbage out." The better you pin down and communicate your main problem(s), the more likely you are to walk out of your doctor's office with the plan that is right for you. Your neurologist is the expert in your disorder, but you and your family are the experts in "you." Physician decision making is not a "one shoe fits all" enterprise, yet when accurate individualized information is lacking, that's what it becomes.

Whether you are startled by hearing a new diagnosis or you come to this knowledge gradually, learning that you have a neurologic problem is jarring. Many neurologic disorders are chronic; you aren't simply adjusting to something new—you will need to deal with this disorder for the foreseeable future. In certain ways, life has changed. Now, there are two crucial "next steps:" the first is finding good neurologic care for your problem, and the second is successfully adjusting to living with your condition. This second step depends upon attaining knowledge of your condition, learning new skills to manage the condition, and finding the flexibility and resourcefulness to restore your quality of life. When successful, you regain your equilibrium and restore a sense of confidence and control that is the cornerstone of well-being.

When healthy adjustment does not occur following a new diagnosis, a sense of feeling out of control and overwhelmed often persists, and no doctor's prescription will adequately respond to this problem. Individuals who acquire good self-management skills are often able to recognize and understand new symptoms and take appropriate action. Conversely, those who are lacking in confidence may respond to the same symptom with a growing sense of anxiety and urgency. In the first case, "watchful waiting" or a call to the physician may result in resolution of the problem. In the second case, the uncertainty and anxiety often leads to multiple physician consultations, unnecessary new prescriptions, social withdrawal, or unwarranted hospitalization. Outcomes can be dramatically different based on knowledge and preparedness.

Managing a neurologic disorder is new territory, and you should not be surprised that you need to be equipped with new information and a new skill set to effectively manage your condition. You will need to learn new words that describe both your symptoms and their treatment to communicate effectively with the members of your medical team. You will also need to learn how to gather accurate information about your condition when you need it and to avoid misinformation. Although each of your physicians document your progress in their medical records, keeping a personal journal about your neurologic condition will help you summarize and track all your medical information in one place. And when you bring this journal with you when you go to see your physician, you will be able to provide more accurate information about your history and previous treatment. Your active and informed involvement in your care and decision making results in a better quality of care and better outcomes.

Your neurologic condition is likely to pose new challenges in daily activities, including interactions in your family, your workplace, and your social and recreational activities. How best can you manage your symptoms or your medication dosing schedule in the context of your normal activities? When should you disclose your diagnosis to others? Neurology Now Books provide you with the background you need, including the experiences of others who have faced similar problems, to guide you through this unfamiliar terrain. Our goal is to give you the resources you need to "take your doctor with you" when you confront these new challenges. We are committed to answering the questions and concerns of individuals living with neurologic disorders and their families in each volume of the Neurology Now Books series. We want you to be as prepared and confident as possible to participate with your doctors in your medical care. Much care is taken to develop each book with you in mind. A special authorship model takes a multidisciplinary team approach to put together the most up-to-date, informative, and useful answers to the questions most concerning you—whether you find yourself in the unexpected role of patient or caregiver. Each authorship team includes neurologists with special expertise, along with a diversity of other contributors with special knowledge of the particular neurologic disorder. Depending upon the specific condition, this includes rehabilitation specialists, nurses, social workers, and people with important shared experiences. Professional writers work to ensure that we avoid "doctor-talk," and easy-to-understand definitions appear on the page when a new term is introduced. Real-life experiences of patients and families are found throughout the text to illustrate important points. And feedback based on correspondence from *Neurology Now* magazine readers informs topics for new books and is integral to our quality improvement. These new features will be found in all books in the Neurology Now Books series, so that you can expect the same quality and patient-centered approach in every volume.

I hope that you have arrived at a new understanding of why "knowledge is empowering" when it comes to your medical care and that Neurology Now Books will serve as an important foundation for the new skills you need to be effective in managing a neurologic condition.

Lisa M. Shulman, MD
Series Editor-in-Chief
Neurology Now Books™

Professor of Neurology
University of Maryland School of Medicine

Acknowledgments

We would like to thank all the people who made this book possible: My wife, Colleen, who spent countless hours reviewing and editing the manuscript; my transcriptionist, Joyce Grein; the staff at the Summit of Lakeway, especially Rose Pera, RN, Carla Powers, and the dining service team headed by Chef Sam Revelles, who helped us conduct our recipe testing with our smell and taste patients; Chris Lee, formerly sous chef at the Four Seasons Hotel in Austin, Texas, for her help developing the first recipes we tested; Dr. David Leake, neuroradiologist at Austin Radiology Associates, for providing copies of MRIs of the brain and CAT scans of the nasal sinuses; Larry Lewis of Projectus, who drew the illustrations for the book; and Jessica Linder, my office manager, who provided some of the recipes and coordinated the patient recipe testing. Special thanks is owed to Richard L. Doty, PhD, Director of the Smell and Taste Center and Professor in the Department of Otorhinolaryngology at the University of Pennsylvania, for taking the time to review the manuscript and offer "spot on" suggestions to improve it, and most of all for writing the foreword. We also want to thank editors Dr. Lisa Shulman and Andrea Weiss, representing the American Academy of Neurology, for their tireless hard work in editing and organizing the subject matter so that the public and health care providers from many disciplines can easily understand and enjoy this book. Finally, journalist Gina Shaw provided valuable expertise in making sure this important topic was relayed as vividly and clearly as possible. Without them this book would not have seen "the light of day."

Introduction

It is hard for many of us to envision a life where we cannot smell and taste our morning coffee or smell a freshly mowed lawn, a bouquet of flowers, or our favorite perfume. Can you imagine not recognizing spoiled food or sour milk—until you taste them and spit them out in disgust? These are only a few examples of life without a normal smell and taste system.

But like the old song says, "You don't know what you've got till it's gone." Many people have no idea just how hard life without the ability to smell and taste normally must be.

If you ask the average person to rate the importance in his or her life of the common senses of hearing, vision, taste, and smell using a number rating system of 1 to 10 in which 1 is least important and 10 most important, the majority would give vision a 10, hearing a 9, and smell and taste a 5. But when you ask people with smell and taste problems the same question, they agree that vision gets a 10 and hearing a 9—but they give smell and taste an 8!

That's because they know that life without a functioning smell and taste system is difficult in many ways:

- ► You may enjoy eating less because food tastes different or has almost no taste at all.
- ► You may not realize when you're in danger from a fire, a gas leak, or spoiled food.
- ► You may have social problems—such as not realizing when you've put on too much perfume or not noticing if you've stepped in a dog mess.
- ► You may have trouble on the job. Imagine a firefighter who can't smell smoke or a chef who can't detect when her soufflé is burning. What about a lineman who doesn't realize he's cut into a gas line?

Could you have a taste or smell disorder? See if you have some of the following common symptoms that are described every day in smell and taste clinics:

- ► Food tastes bland.
- ► Everything tastes the same.

> ► Eating isn't enjoyable.
> ► Every time I eat, I get a bad taste in my mouth.

Did you notice something about this list? Almost no one mentions the sense of smell. Most people with smell and taste disorders are most distressed about their absent or altered sense of taste. They notice that they do not smell as well as they used to—frequently, they cannot smell anything—but problems with taste are usually what people find most troubling. But, in fact, the two senses are closely linked; usually, if you have a problem with one, you have a problem with the other as well. The majority of people who have taste symptoms really have a problem with their sense of smell. A normal smell and taste system is necessary for you to recognize flavors. If either system is impaired—more so with smell—you will likely have difficulty recognizing flavors.

Smell and taste disorders become more common as we age. As many as 14 million Americans over age 55 have smell impairment. Some studies have shown that half of people between 65 and 80 and three-fourths of people over 80 have smell and taste problems. Since Americans are living longer and longer lives, more and more will develop smell and taste difficulties.

Smell loss may affect 14 million people over age 55.

If you are reading this book, you are probably one of them—and so am I. One day in 1995, I noticed that the milk on my breakfast cereal tasted very sour. Although I have the habit of smelling the milk carton, I hadn't detected that the milk had gone bad. I realized that I could not smell the sour milk. A few days later, while cleaning out the dog pen, I noticed that the dog's stool smelled sweet rather than foul. That part wasn't a problem, although I did get stuck with full-time dog cleanup as a result. But I knew my sense of smell had changed, and I decided I needed to learn more about why.

After spending time with Dr. Richard L. Doty, director of the Smell and Taste Center at the University of Pennsylvania in Philadelphia and a pioneer in smell and taste disorders, I eventually developed my own Taste and Smell Disorders Clinic as part of my neurology practice in Austin, Texas. Since establishing this practice in 1996, I have observed a great deal of progress in understanding, diagnosing, and treating smell and taste disorders.

These developments include standardized smell testing, improved taste testing, and major advances in imaging, particularly computed tomography (CT) and magnetic resonance imaging (MRI). In addition, major advances have also been made in our knowledge at the cellular and genetic levels. Indeed, in 2004, the Nobel Prize was awarded for the first time to scientists in the field of smell and taste, Dr. Richard Axel and Dr. Linda Buck. They discovered the genes for the first of many olfactory receptors (of which you will learn more about in Chapter 1), and found that they are very diverse. These developments have allowed us to better understand the natural history of smell and taste changes in the normal aging population and in disorders of smell and taste.

During the past 20 years, clinical research trials have uncovered disorders of smell and taste in people with Parkinson's disease and multiple sclerosis, as well as certain dementias like Alzheimer's disease and Lewy body disease—disorders that had previously often gone unrecognized because people with these conditions often do not report that they are having difficulties with smell or taste. During the course of these illnesses, decreased appetite, weight loss, and depression often occur, which may be falsely attributed to other disorders. In fact, currently some evidence indicates that smell testing in the normal population has been of some help in predicting who may later develop cognitive impairment, Alzheimer's disease, or Parkinson's disease.

Since the early years of the twenty-first century, ongoing long-term follow-up studies of the population with impaired smell and taste disorders have shown that many of these disorders improve with time, an encouraging finding that was not well recognized or appreciated in the past.

Unfortunately, most of this information hasn't reached the average doctor's office, and it is one of the main reasons for writing this book, which will guide you through the subject of smell and taste. This book will help you understand why the smell and taste system does not always work properly—for example, in my case, my smell disorder was caused by a cold virus (about one in four smell disorders are due to viral infections). This book will also tell you how these conditions affect our daily lives, and probably what you're most interested in: how we can cope with them, and what we can do to treat some of these conditions, including a special section featuring modified recipes and guidelines for food preparation that can make a big difference in how much you enjoy your meals.

Navigating
Smell and **Taste**
Disorders

Why Can't I Smell?

In this chapter, you'll learn:

▶ The most common causes of smell disorders

▶ Symptoms of smell disorders

▶ How smell disorders can sometimes alert physicians to other neurologic conditions, such as Alzheimer's disease or Parkinson's disease

Andrew, a 40-year-old truck driver, was stopped at a red light when another driver rear-ended him. He escaped the accident with only a mild bruise and checked out fine in the emergency department. But four days later, Andrew began to notice something strange. First, his morning coffee smelled flat. Next, he filled up his truck and found that he couldn't smell the powerful odor of the diesel gasoline. What had happened? Was something wrong with his nose?

Like Andrew, many people develop smell disorders after being injured in an accident. But the most common cause of smell disorders is something none of us can avoid: normal aging.

Common Causes of Smell Disorders

Normal aging causes the majority of smell disorders. Two-thirds of the remaining problems with chronic smell loss are due to upper respiratory tract infections (colds), head trauma, and disorders of the

Common Causes of Smell Disorders

► Normal aging

► Disorders of nasal passages and sinuses (examples: sinusitis, nasal polyps, nasal cancer)

► Viral infections of the nose and upper airway (examples: common cold, influenza)

► Head and nose injuries

► Medications

► Toxins

► Smoking

► Alcohol

► Chronic medical disorders

► Neurologic disorders

► Psychiatric disorders

► Congenital anosmia (smell disorder from birth)

nasal passages and sinuses. Other causes may include many prescribed medications, thyroid and vitamin deficiency, diabetes, and various neurologic disorders such as Alzheimer's disease and Parkinson's disease.

Normal Aging

Normal aging is the most common cause of loss of smell or taste. Smell loss occurs in:

► 2 percent of the normal population under 65
► 50 percent of the population between 65 and 80
► 75 percent of the population over age 80

It is more common in men than in women because women generally lose their sense of smell later than men. In fact, women of all ages do better than men in smell testing.

But not all smells are impaired with aging. Surprisingly—for reasons we do not understand—certain smells such as chocolate, licorice, rose, strawberry, watermelon, coconut, and natural grass show little or no change as we age.

The vast majority of older adults who have a smell disorder do not fully realize that they have a problem. They may recognize that their food does not taste the same, but they usually do not know that the culprit is probably an impaired sense of smell interfering with their ability to recognize flavors. Particularly for older people, it is very important to properly recognize, diagnose, and manage smell disorders, since the loss of the sense of smell may lead to poor appetite, unhealthy weight loss, and malnourishment.

Why does our sense of smell change as we age? There are several causes, including:

▶ A reduced number of olfactory nerve cells **(olfactory receptors)**.
▶ Closing of the **cribriform plate**, the bony openings where the olfactory nerves enter the inside of the skull on their way to the brain. The closing of these bony openings pinch off the olfactory nerve fibers and reduces their number.
▶ Less blood flow in the nasal **smell organ**, which is made up of specialized sensory cells found high within the nasal cavity.
▶ Increased thickness of nasal mucus.

Disorders of the Nasal Passages and Sinuses

Fifty-eight-year-old Grace was relieved when she finally began to recover from the stubborn cold that had plagued her for more than a week. Her cough, sniffles, fever, and general achiness began to subside. But just as she was feeling better, she discovered a new problem: her food tasted bland and flavorless. She got into the shower one morning and noticed that her Tahitian coconut shower gel smelled neither Tahitian nor like coconut. She was completely over her cold in a few days, but as the months went on, her sense of smell did not return. Grace's appetite decreased, and she no longer enjoyed her favorite meals since she could not smell or taste her food.

Olfactory receptors Nerve cells (neurons) in the nasal smell organ that are responsible for receiving and transmitting information about smell. They are the largest family in the human genome.

Cribriform plate A bone in the front of the skull directly above the smell organ in the nose. It has many tiny holes through which the olfactory nerve fibers travel to reach the inside of the skull.

Smell organ Located high up in the nasal cavity and made up of specialized nerve cells called olfactory cells. The main function of these cells is to identify odors and recognize different flavors.

Like Grace, many people develop smell disorders as a result of common ailments that we all get: colds, sinus infections, allergies (such as allergic **rhinitis**—commonly known as a runny nose), and nasal polyps. These conditions can cause smell disorders for different reasons. For example, they can partially or completely block the nasal passages, preventing odor molecules from reaching the smell organ.

When you have a particularly bad cold, in between feeling miserable with sniffling, sneezing, and coughing, you might notice that food doesn't smell or taste as appetizing as usual. This is because of swelling and congestion of the nasal passages. Most of the time, your sense of smell returns to normal when your cold goes away—but not always.

Viruses cause about one-quarter of all cases of permanent (partial or complete) smell loss. Certain viruses are particularly likely to cause chronic smell loss; one of these is the parainfluenza virus, which causes respiratory tract infections. The virus may damage the nerve cells of the smell organ or the **olfactory bulbs** beneath the brain. This occurs more commonly in women than in men and usually occurs in people over 55. Partial loss of smell is more common than total loss of smell.

Nearly two-thirds of people who have smell loss from viral infections develop **dysosmia**, a distorted sense of smell that is usually unpleasant. Dysosmia happens as a result of damage to some of the olfactory nerve receptor cells. The bad smell may occur out of the blue or be triggered by other everyday odors. One-third of people will also report an altered taste because damage to the olfactory nerve cells—from a viral illness or any other cause—can lead to inability to appreciate and recognize flavors.

Chances for recovery are unpredictable. In general, the more severe the smell loss, the less certain the chance of recovery. Recovery usually begins in the first six months, with the greatest chance of recovery during the first two years. About two-thirds of cases of virus-related smell loss improve over three to four years. When biopsies are per-

---

Rhinitis Irritation and inflammation of some areas of the lining of the nose. Commonly described as a runny nose.

Olfactory bulb Located in the front or base of the brain (the forebrain), the olfactory bulb is where the olfactory nerves from the smell organ in the nose end and the olfactory tracts within the brain begin.

Dysosmia The perception of a smell, usually unpleasant, that may be triggered by a normal smell or arise without a known trigger.

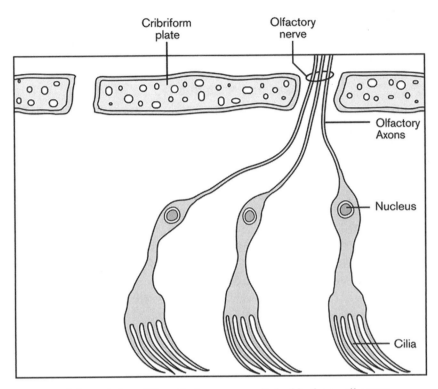

Figure 1   Enlarged view of the olfactory nerve cells inside the smell organ.

formed to look at the smell organ under a microscope, doctors have found that many of the olfactory nerve cells are missing, and the cells that are present have lost their **cilia** and axons (see Figure 1), which send smell signals to and from the cells.

Allergies with inflammation may also damage the nerve cells involved in smell. Most of these disorders are easily treated and reversible with decongestants, nasal sprays, or nasal and sinus surgery. Despite treatment, a *few* continue to have smell loss due to damage of

---

Cilia Microscopic hairs found within the nasal smell organ (different from the larger nose hairs found near the opening of the nostril). These tiny hairs, bathed in the mucous of the nose, project from the olfactory receptor cells, capturing odors as they enter the nose and beginning the process of transmitting the odors to the brain.

the olfactory nerve cells. An ear, nose, and throat specialist often treats these disorders. Chronic nasal allergies can also be diagnosed and treated by allergists and immunologists.

About two-thirds of cases of virus-related smell loss improve over three to four years.

Head and Nose Injuries

Smell and taste problems are reported in about one-tenth of all head injuries—even those as mild as Andrew's, the truck driver from the beginning of this chapter, who had only a little bruising and a headache after being rear-ended. But they increase to nearly two-thirds when the injuries are more severe, such as when a skull fracture occurs. Two-thirds of people with severe head injuries have total smell loss, and one-third have partial or no smell loss.

Head and nose injuries that lead to smell and taste problems usually occur in accidents involving falls: crashes of bicycles, motorcycles, or motor vehicles and injuries from sports, such as boxing, football, and soccer.

Head injuries can result in damage to the smell system in a number of different ways:

▶ Direct injury to the nose and head, which damages the smell organ and the nerves that travel through the bones of the upper nose and base of the skull.

▶ Injury to the olfactory bulb and nerves inside the skull.

▶ Injury to the **temporal** and **frontal lobes** of the brain, which receive messages from the smell organ and are involved in the recognition of odors. The base of the skull has very rough interior edges and ridges, and movement of the brain along the base of the skull during the injury can cause bruising of the temporal and frontal lobes.

Studies show that injuries to the back and sides of the head are more likely to cause smell loss than injuries to the front of the head. This is because there is more cartilage in the front of the head and nose, which

Temporal lobe There are two temporal lobes, one on each side of the brain located at about the level of the ears in the temporal region of the skull. The temporal lobes play an important role in speech, memory, hearing, and identification and recognition of odors.

Frontal lobe The front one-third of the brain. It is very important in our ability to reason, plan, judge, have insight, be attentive, behave appropriately, and recognize and identify everyday odors.

tends to absorb the impact of a crash or fall better than the back and sides of the head.

There is no specific treatment for smell loss from head and nose injuries. Injuries to the smell organ may heal over time after the swelling and bruising in the nose heals. Injuries to the olfactory nerves in the nose and brain usually improve with time, but not completely. Studies show that two years following head injury, about one-third of patients had their smell impairment improve slightly, one-fifth worsened, and nearly half remained the same. A 2008 study[1] that followed people with smell loss for many years—longer than any other such research—suggests that improvement and recovery of smell function depend upon the age of the person and the severity of the smell loss (which can be determined by testing, as explained in Chapter 4). These two factors are much more important predictors of recovery than the actual cause of the smell loss. Mild to moderate smell loss after head trauma has an excellent chance of improving. Dysosmia (the perception of a foul odor that is not actually there) is common in these cases and always improves, although in some it may take years.

Researchers are currently looking for new approaches to trigger regeneration of the **olfactory system** following injury. Scientists are studying the use of medications or cell transplantation to replace the injured olfactory nerve cells.[1] It is hoped that this ongoing research will be successful so that more people will recover following smell loss.

> Mild to moderate smell loss after head trauma has a good chance of improving.

Medications

Caroline had been plagued by painful migraines ever since she was a teenager. In her mid-forties, the medications that once helped to manage her headaches seemed to become less effective, so her doctor switched her to a combination of two new drugs, diltiazem (Cardizem, Dilacor, Tiazac), which also helped to control her mild high blood pressure, and topiramate (Topamax). Soon both her migraines and her blood pressure had improved. But about a month later, Caroline pulled a cold can of cola out of the refrigerator, opened it, and took a long gulp—only to make a face because the soda tasted flat and unpleasant. The next morning as she was brewing a fresh pot of coffee, she realized that she could barely smell the pungent beans. And as she and her

---

Olfactory system The nasal smell organ, olfactory bulb, tracts, and olfactory cortex.

husband prepared to go out to dinner one night, he pulled her aside and told her that she might want to wear just a little less Chanel No. 5.

A wide variety of medications, many of them commonly used, can cause smell and taste problems. Medications can affect smell by changing nasal secretions and nasal blood flow or by preventing normal electrical discharges of the smell receptors.

Some of the medications that most commonly cause smell loss include:

- ▶ Antihistamines: chlorpheniramine maleate (common in decongestants and cough syrups)
- ▶ Antibiotics: penicillin(s) and tetracycline(s)
- ▶ Cold prevention: zinc gluconate gel (nasal spray)
- ▶ Blood pressure medications: diltiazem (Cardizem, Dilacor, Tiazac) and nifedipine (Procardia, Procardia XL, Adalat CC)
- ▶ Cholesterol-lowering drugs: atorvastatin (Lipitor) and pravastatin (Pravachol)
- ▶ Narcotics: codeine and morphine
- ▶ Chemotherapy drugs: methotrexate
- ▶ Amphetamines
- ▶ Local anesthetics: cocaine
- ▶ Stomach acid drugs: cimetidine (Tagamet)
- ▶ Antidepressants: amitriptyline (Elavil, Vanatrip) and paroxetine (Paxil)
- ▶ Antiseizure: phenytoin (Dilantin)
- ▶ Diuretics: furosemide (Lasix)

In 2003, hundreds of people who used the nasal sprays Cold-Eze and Zicam, both cold remedies of zinc gluconate gel, sued the manufacturers of these sprays after developing smell loss. They shared a common story: shortly after using the zinc nasal spray to prevent or shorten a cold, the users felt a burning sensation in their nose. Within 24 hours or less, they experienced a loss of smell and resulting disturbances in taste. This phenomenon probably resulted from stimulation of the sensory part of the **trigeminal nerve** (Figure 2). In most people

---

Trigeminal nerve Also called the fifth cranial nerve. It carries information about touch, temperature, and pain to the brain from the face and inside the mouth, tongue, and teeth. It also carries information about texture, temperature, and spiciness of food and sends this information to the brain.

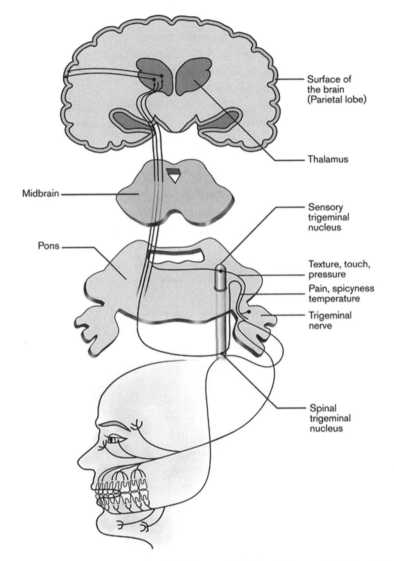

Figure 2   Sensory nerve supply of the face and inside of the mouth by the fifth cranial nerve (trigeminal) and its pathway to the brain.

with this condition described in medical literature, little or no improvement has occurred after one year. Longer follow-up studies will be necessary to see if this smell loss is permanent. However, thousands of people have used this nasal spray without incident. The manufacturer of Cold-Eze has since stopped making the spray, while Zicam remained on the market until June 2009. Its manufacturer, Matrixx, settled a class-action lawsuit brought by 340 Zicam users who claimed a loss of smell for $12 million in 2005. As it is a homeopathic remedy, it is unregulated by the U.S. Food and Drug Administration (FDA). In the spring of 2009, the FDA recommended to the manufacturer that they voluntarily remove Zicam nasal gel and swabs from the market because of their potential to cause severe smell loss. The manufacturer is currently following the FDA recommendations. Zicam is still available and appears to be safe in rapid-dissolving and chewable tablets.

Despite the settlement of the lawsuit and removal of the product from the market, it is still unclear whether the smell loss experienced was due to the Zicam products or to the cold virus.

Toxins

People who have been exposed to toxins such as pesticides, formaldehyde, carbon disulfides, and sulfuric acid—often during the course of their jobs—may experience smell loss as a result. Toxins may interfere with smell by causing inflammation (swelling) that blocks the nasal pathway or by damaging the olfactory receptors. Brief exposure to most of these toxins may result in temporary smell loss with good recovery. However, some toxins, like sulfur dioxide and cresol powder, may cause permanent smell loss.

Smoking

As you'll learn in Chapter 5, one of the ways Andrew, the truck driver who experienced smell loss after a car accident, regained some of his sense of smell was by quitting smoking, something he was persuaded to do by the staff at the taste and smell clinic he visited. It has been known since the 1980s that smoking causes smell loss; it also can make smell loss from other causes, such as trauma or age-related smell loss, significantly worse. Secondhand smoke may also cause smell loss. One study showed children of smoking parents scored 10 percent lower on smell tests than children of nonsmoking parents. How smoking causes smell loss is not clear. It seems likely that chemicals in the smoke affect the olfactory receptor cells and mucous lining of the smell organ.

A 1990 study suggested that heavy smokers (one-and-a-half to two packs per day) who quit, regain some of their smell function over time.[2] The bad news is that the recovery time is very slow, and it may even take as long as the number of years the person smoked. The good news is that the amount of smell loss from smoking is generally small.

Alcohol

Alcoholism has many health consequences, including injury to the liver and nervous system. In the 1970s, researchers found that people with alcoholism had difficulty with odor identification and odor memory. In 2003, a study showed that about half of chronic drinkers had difficulty identifying odors.[3]

What is the cause of smell loss in chronic drinkers? The evidence suggests that the problem is in the brain's olfactory system rather than in the nasal smell organ or the olfactory bulbs. The brain regions that are affected are the **prefrontal** and **orbital frontal lobes**, which are both important for smell function. (See Chapter 3 for more details on how these elements of our smell and taste system work together in the perception of smell and taste.) These brain regions are also important in controlling emotions and behavior, and in reasoning and decision making. Fortunately, when people stop drinking excessively, their smell function may improve.

Chronic Medical Disorders

A host of familiar medical disorders can last for many years despite available treatments. Some of these more common medical conditions can alter smell and taste; they include low thyroid function, diabetes, and liver and kidney diseases.

Having a low level of thyroid hormone (called hypothyroidism) can lessen sensitivity to smell and taste. When thyroid function returns to normal (usually after the use of thyroid medication), smell and taste usually returns to normal as well. However, about one-fifth of people continue to have a burning mouth sensation and an unpleasant taste even after their thyroid condition is corrected. The

---

Prefrontal lobe The front part of the frontal lobe, the part of the forebrain, involved in reasoning, decision making, and controlling emotions.

Orbital frontal lobe The front part of the frontal lobe that sits directly above the orbit (eye socket) of the inside of the skull. This part of the brain allows us to appreciate and develop emotional connections to odors.

cause is unknown, but it may be a combination of changes in saliva and changes of the smell and taste nerve cells and their connections in the brain.

Half of all people with diabetes experience problems with smell and taste. They are less sensitive to common odors and tastes, especially sugar. The cause is unknown. However, diabetics frequently experience nerve damage throughout the body, known as neuropathy. (The most common is **peripheral neuropathy**, which causes numbness in the hands and feet.) It is possible that smell and taste changes in diabetics are due to neuropathy affecting the smell and taste nerves.

People who have altered kidney function for long periods of time can develop smell and taste impairment, resulting in less sensitivity to common smells and tastes. This is likely due to multiple factors, which include medications used to treat the kidney disorder, low zinc levels that may develop, and the kidney disease itself, which can lead to abnormal accumulation of some body waste products and alter smell and taste nerve cells and their connections to the brain. Improvement in kidney function with medications and dialysis usually results in improved smell and taste. In some cases, changes in medications are necessary. A blood test can determine the zinc level, and, if it is low, zinc supplements should be recommended.

Two-thirds of people with chronic liver disease (cirrhosis) have smell and taste loss. Liver disease can be caused by many things, such as viral hepatitis, liver injury from accidents, cancer, and heavy alcohol use. Similarly to kidney disease, when liver disease results in smell and taste loss, it is probably because of failure of the liver to remove many of the body's waste products. The more impaired the liver function, the more smell and taste symptoms there are. Medications used to treat liver disease may also play a role. When liver function improves, smell and taste generally improve as well.

Neurologic Disorders

Neurologic disorders such as Alzheimer's disease, Parkinson's disease, frontotemporal dementia, and multiple sclerosis may interfere with smell and taste function. People with these diseases, and the family

---

Peripheral neuropathy Damage to the peripheral nervous system, the nerves that send information from the limbs back to the spinal cord and brain. Symptoms include numbness and tingling and weakness in the hands and feet.

and friends who care for them, may notice that they have reduced appetite, less interest in food, and weight loss, but they may not realize the cause. Doctors may attribute these symptoms to medications or other illnesses, especially since the patient—particularly one with dementia—often does not report problems with his or her sense of smell or taste. When asked directly, however, many people with these disorders tell us that they have less interest and enjoyment in eating because food doesn't taste the same.

Alzheimer's Disease

Alzheimer's disease is the most common cause of dementia in people aged 65 and older. Alzheimer's disease is a cognitive disorder that interferes with memory, insight, and judgment. Other problems include word-finding difficulty and personality changes.

During the mid-1980s, researchers found that the olfactory system, which consists of the nasal smell organ, olfactory bulb, and parts of the brain, is impaired in Alzheimer's disease from very early on and worsens over time. Smell loss occurs in Alzheimer's disease because nerve cells

> **Ninety percent of people with Alzheimer's disease have a progressive— and usually unrecognized— smell disorder.**

in the olfactory system are damaged. Studies show problems with smell function in 90 percent of people with Alzheimer's disease. Still, the majority of people with Alzheimer's do not report noticing problems with their smell.

Recently, it has been discovered that people with **mild cognitive impairment (MCI)**, a mild form of memory loss that is often a precursor to Alzheimer's disease, are more likely to develop dementia if they have abnormal smell function on a smell test—especially if it includes the 10 odors most likely to be impaired in Alzheimer's. These 10 odors are menthol, clove, leather, strawberry, lilac, pineapple, smoke, soap, natural gas, and lemon. Another study has shown that an abnormal smell

Alzheimer's disease The most common cause of dementia in people aged 65 and older; a progressive cognitive disorder that interferes with memory, insight, and judgment.

Mild cognitive impairment (MCI) A mild form of memory loss that is often a precursor to Alzheimer's disease and other dementias.

test score on the University of Pennsylvania smell identification test of 32/40 or less in people with MCI predicts a greater thsan 60 percent likelihood of developing Alzheimer disease.[4]

Eighty to 90 percent of people with Parkinson's disease have moderate smell loss.

Parkinson's Disease and Related Disorders

Parkinson's disease is a movement disorder characterized by resting tremor of one or both arms and legs, rigidity (stiffness), slowing of movements, and problems with walking and balance. Between 80 and 90 percent of people with Parkinson's show moderate smell loss when tested. A recent smell study identified five odors commonly unrecognized in Parkinson's disease: gasoline, banana, pineapple, smoke, and cinnamon.

The reason for smell loss in this disorder is because an abnormal substance called **alpha-synuclein** builds up in the nasal smell organ, olfactory bulb, and parts of the brain, resulting in injury to nerve cells.

People with Parkinson's disease have also been found to sniff less frequently than the average person, which contributes to smell loss. Sniffing is part of our normal smell process, which helps identify odors. When people with Parkinson's disease sniff, it is very shallow compared to normal sniffing, and less air and odors reach the smell organ. Smell loss in Parkinson's disease does not appear to get worse over time as it does in Alzheimer's disease. It is also not associated with the duration of Parkinson's disease or Parkinson's medications. The maximum amount of smell loss occurs early in the disease process—in fact, usually earlier than the common Parkinson's symptoms of tremor or slowness of movement. As with Alzheimer's disease, smell problems may also be a predictor of increased risk of Parkin-

---

Parkinson's disease A movement disorder characterized by resting tremor of one or both arms and legs, rigidity (stiffness), slowing of movements, and problems with walking and balance.

Alpha-synuclein A protein found in normal nerve cells. Its function remains unknown. It is abnormal and appears to be the source for smell loss when it accumulates in the olfactory bulb, tracts, and medial temporal lobe, which is the area of the brain that stores personal memories, general knowledge and facts, and recognizes odors. It is often found in people with Parkinson's disease and related disorders.

son's disease. When close relatives of Parkinson's patients were evaluated for smell loss it was found that the presence of smell loss was associated with a 25 percent risk of developing Parkinson's disease over the next two years.

People with Lewy body disease, a neurologic disorder that combines mild tremors and other Parkinson-like symptoms with confusion and visual hallucinations, also have moderate to severe smell impairment. Smell testing may also help to differentiate Parkinson's disease from other related neurologic disorders that may be easily confused with Parkinson's but are not associated with smell loss. For example, people with a condition known as familial or essential tremor usually have normal smell on testing. Although this condition involves arm movement only, with no stiffness or balance problems, it can frequently be mistaken for Parkinson's. (The movie star Katharine Hepburn had this condition, which caused her to have a head and voice tremor.)

Frontotemporal Dementia
Frontotemporal dementia, the third most common type of dementia after Alzheimer's disease and dementia related to Parkinson's disease, usually begins with changes in personality and childlike behavior. Unlike Alzheimer's disease, memory usually remains normal in the early stages of the disease and declines later. It has recently been determined that up to 70 percent of people with frontotemporal dementia have smell loss, with a smell impairment similar to that found in people with Alzheimer's disease. It is not clear if their smell loss worsens with time. Unlike with Alzheimer's and Parkinson's diseases, the olfactory receptors, bulb, and tracts are normal in this condition; instead, it appears that abnormalities in the frontal lobe and temporal lobe of the brain may be responsible for smell loss.

Multiple Sclerosis
Multiple sclerosis (MS) is usually diagnosed between the ages of 15 and 50, occurs more commonly in women, and affects the function of the brain and spinal cord. Symptoms, which include numbness,

---

Multiple sclerosis (MS) A neurologic disorder of the brain and spinal cord of unknown cause. It usually affects individuals between 15 and 50 years of age. Symptoms usually come and go but can be progressive. Symptoms include visual loss, numbness or weakness of one or more limbs, and poor balance.

weakness, and visual loss, have a tendency to come and go. Attacks of MS are associated with the development of **plaques** (abnormal scar tissue from inflammation that accumulates between nerve cells) in the brain and spinal cord that can be seen on **magnetic resonance imaging (MRI)**. MRI is a special x-ray that aligns hydrogen molecules of water present in body tissue by a powerful magnet and leads to good images of the tissues studied. Under the microscope, these plaques show inflammation, swelling, and loss of the protective coating called myelin that covers the nerve fibers. These plaques may occur in areas of the brain that represent smell and taste functions.

Twenty to 30 percent of people with MS have mild to moderate smell loss on testing. The degree of smell loss is associated with the number of MS plaques in the temporal and frontal lobes of the brain, the areas that are responsible for the recognition of odors. Nonetheless, only 5 percent of MS patients with smell loss are actually aware of it.[5] Since MS attacks and plaques in the brain can come and go, smell test results can also fluctuate.[6] In rare situations, taste changes may be the first symptom of a MS flare-up. These taste changes usually last a short time.

Seizures

Seizure disorders occur in 2 percent of the population, and they are caused by abnormal electrical discharges in the brain. Some people with seizure disorders experience an **aura**—an unusual sen-

---

Plaques Abnormal deposits of protein between nerve cells in the brain. These deposits can be made up of a protein called beta-amyloid, and are characteristic of Alzheimer's disease. Plaques of a different kind occur in multiple sclerosis. These plaques are areas of inflammation and scarring due to damage of the covering of nerve fibers in the brain and spinal cord.

Magnetic resonance imaging (MRI) A medical imaging technique used to visualize the body's internal structure and function. It provides contrast between the different soft tissues of the body, using a powerful magnetic field rather than the radiation that is used in computed tomographic (or CT) scans and x-rays.

Aura An unusual sensation, sense of dread, or hallucination experienced by some people with seizure disorders before the seizure begins. This term is used to describe a phenomenon experienced by some people at the beginning of a migraine headache. The term visual or sensory aura is used when a person with migraine develops either flashing lights or numbness and tingling before a headache begins.

sation, sense of dread, or hallucination–before the seizure begins. Some auras are visual, such as flashing lights; but about 15 percent of all auras involve smell or taste, with smell auras occurring more frequently.

Smell auras are usually unpleasant, like that of burning rubber or rotten eggs. These auras are usually brief, lasting less than two minutes. MRI scans of the temporal lobes, in which the brain smell center lies and where these abnormal electrical discharges occur, may find the cause of the olfactory auras. Causes may include brain tumors, cysts, aneurysms, strokes, and brain injury. Auras usually improve with the use of antiseizure medication.

Smell auras are very different from dysosmia. Dysosmia refers to an usually unpleasant smell that lasts much longer than an aura of a seizure, from more than two minutes to several hours. Seizure auras usually last less than two minutes, usually 30 to 45 seconds. Dysosmia can either be triggered by a normal everyday smell, or develop out of the blue. It is usually caused by abnormal function of the olfactory organ in the nose or olfactory bulb and tracts inside the skull, not the brain.

Migraine

About 60 percent of people who have severe headaches have migraines, a specific headache disorder of unknown cause that can present itself in at least three different ways. The classic migraine involves spots or light flashes in the vision, followed by nausea or vomiting and a severe, throbbing, one-sided headache that usually requires the person to lie down in a dark room.

Another common type of migraine is a gradually increasing throbbing headache, with or without nausea and sensitivity to light. This type may or may not require the person to lie down in a dark room.

A third type of migraine involves the development of spots or lights in the eyes for five minutes or more; these visual disturbances subside without a headache.

Smell symptoms have been recognized for a long time in people with migraine. Migraine patients will often say that their migraine attacks are triggered by certain odors. The triggers most commonly reported are strong perfume and gasoline. Twenty-five percent of participants in a 2004 research study reported that their attack was triggered by a strong odor; most of those reporting this trigger were women.[7] Spontaneous bad smells (phantosmia) can also replace spots and flashing lights as part of a migraine aura or warning, although this is rare—probably involving less than 1 percent of migraine patients. Many people with migraines also report that everyday smells can make their headaches worse.

Psychiatric Disorders

Schizophrenia is a serious psychiatric disorder that causes disturbances in thinking, perception, and emotions. Smell loss occurs in 50 percent of people with this disorder.[8] It begins early in the disease process and worsens over time. Men and women are equally affected. One-third of healthy family members of schizophrenic patients also have smell loss on testing, suggesting a possible genetic link. The cause of this smell loss is due to a disturbance of olfactory processing in the **olfactory cortex** (surface) of the frontal and temporal lobes of the brain, which are responsible for the conscious awareness and identification of odors.

Congenital Anosmia

Congenital anosmia is the inability to smell odors from the time of birth. It is unknown exactly how often this occurs. MRI scans of the brain show absence or incomplete development of the olfactory bulbs and tracts, structures located in the front of the base of the brain that relay smell signals. This appears to be a dominant genetic disorder, which means that a child born to someone with congenital anosmia has a fifty-fifty chance of having the same disorder. People with congenital anosmia do not report smell or taste problems because they are not aware of the normal smells and tastes of everyday life. No specific treatment is known. It is important for people with this disorder to be educated. Safety concerns related to smell loss need to be emphasized, including problems with detecting smoke or recognizing spoiled foods.

Schizophrenia A serious psychiatric disorder that causes disturbances in thinking, perception, and emotions.

Olfactory cortex This term refers to parts of the brain that receive smell information. It includes a number of different brain structures: the deep inner side of the temporal lobe and the amygdala (a structure deep in the temporal lobe). The olfactory cortex is responsible for odor identification and intensity, not the ability to detect an odor.

Congenital anosmia Complete absence of the sense of smell from birth.

References

1. London B, Nabet B, Fisher AR, et al. Predictors of prognosis in patients with olfactory disturbance. *Annals of Neurology* 2008;63(2):159–166.

This article describes the common causes of smell loss but is especially important because the authors followed some of the patients for over 23 years, making this one of the longest studies ever reported. This study, therefore, provides a really accurate picture of the outcome of smell loss due to different causes.

2. Frye RE, Schwartz BS, Doty RI. Dose-related effects of cigarette smoking on olfactory function. *JAMA* 1990;263(9):1233–1236.

This study followed smokers for many years and gives an interesting picture of how smoking interferes with smell and taste in the long term. Even though the article was written 20 years ago, it remains an excellent source on this important subject.

3. Rupp C, Kurz M, Kemmler G, et al. Olfactory sensitivity, discrimination, and identification in patients with alcohol dependence. *Journal of Alcoholism: Clinical and Experimental Research* 2003;27(3):432–439.

The authors of this article have a vast experience in alcohol-related smell loss. This is one of their excellent published papers on the subject.

4. Devanand DP, Michaels-Marston KS, Liu X, et al. Olfactory deficits in patients with mild cognitive impairment predicts Alzheimer's disease at follow-up. *American Journal of Psychiatry* 2000;157(9):1399–1405.

This paper describes a large population with mild cognitive impairment who are given the UPSIT smell test and followed for a number of years. Individuals who scored 32/40 or less initially had over a 50 percent probability of converting to early Alzheimer's disease. It is important to note than any person with mild cognitive impairment has a significant risk of getting worse over a five-year period and converting to Alzheimer's dementia. A positive smell test, as described in this article, helps predict to whom this is more likely to happen.

5. Doty RL, Li C, Mannon LJ, et al. Olfactory dysfunction in multiple sclerosis: relation to longitudinal changes in plaque numbers in central olfactory structures. *Neurology* 1999;53(4):880–882.

This study of a group of patients with multiple sclerosis (MS) showed that smell loss is related to the number of areas of inflammation and scarring caused by MS in the smell centers of the frontal and temporal lobe. This study helped explain why many patients with MS have normal smell, since MS plaques can occur anywhere in the brain, not always just in the smell center.

6. Doty RL, Li C, Mannon LJ, et al. Olfactory dysfunction in multiple sclerosis. Relation to plaque load in inferior frontal and temporal lobes. *Annuals of the New York Academy Of Sciences* 1998;30(855):781–786.

This study was the first to show that smell test results can vary in people with multiple sclerosis, improving when both attacks and inflammation in the smell centers of the frontal and temporal lobe subside.

7. Kelman L. The premonitory symptoms (prodrome): a tertiary care study of 893 migraineurs. *Headache* 2004;44(9):865–872.

This paper studied one of the largest groups of people with migraine to see how common and what kinds of auras or symptoms occurred before the development of headaches. Because of the large number of patients studied, it gives us very reliable information on this subject.

8. Kopala LC, Good KP, Morrison K, et al. Impaired olfactory identification in relatives of patients with familial schizophrenia. *American Journal of Psychiatry* 2001;158(8):1286–1290.

This study followed a large number of people with schizophrenia, relatives with and without schizophrenia, and a group of unrelated healthy people. Smell testing was done on all of them.

The study found that half of those with schizophrenia and one-third of family members without schizophrenia had mild smell impairment. Only 9 percent of the healthy control population had a mild smell loss. This study suggested that genetic factors appear to possibly be playing a role in smell impairment in schizophrenia.

2

Why Can't I Taste?

In this chapter, you'll learn:

▶ The most common causes of taste disorders
▶ Symptoms of taste disorders
▶ Common medical terms used in discussing taste disorders

Over a period of two weeks, Genevieve, a 55-year-old woman with diabetes and hypertension, began noticing a bizarre taste in her mouth. The sweet, metallic flavor never seemed to go away, except when she ate. When she chewed foods, she could still appreciate the tartness of a Granny Smith apple or the savory taste of roast beef. (Her sense of smell was unaffected.) Soon she found herself eating almost constantly to avoid the bad taste. Genevieve's weight began to skyrocket, and her diabetes and hypertension became harder to control.

Genevieve was an unusual patient—her taste disorder had nothing to do with her sense of smell. Nine out of ten people who have taste symptoms actually have a smell problem. This is because the smell system is more vulnerable than the taste system. There is just one small smell organ and one **cranial nerve** to transmit smell information while the

---

Cranial nerves Twelve paired nerves (one for each side of the body) that emerge directly from the brain stem, primarily serving the motor and sensory systems of the head and neck.

Common Medical Terms Used When Discussing Taste Disorders

When you see your doctor or read about taste disorders, you will most likely encounter a number of specific medical words and phrases. The following are the most common medical terms used. They are all derived from the Greek word *geusi*, which means "taste."

Ageusia Total loss of taste.

Hypogeusia Partial loss of taste.

Hypergeusia Increased sense of taste. Regular tastes, such as sweet or sour, appear unusually powerful.

Dysgeusia The presence of an altered taste, usually unpleasant.

Parageusia A usually unpleasant taste triggered by another taste.

Phantageusia A usually unpleasant taste that arises out of the blue.

taste system has many taste receptors and multiple connections to the brain (you'll learn more about this in Chapter 4). With impaired smell function, your ability to identify and appreciate flavors is limited, even if your taste function is normal. It is uncommon to have a smell disorder without it affecting your taste as well, but, as Genevieve's case shows, the opposite is not true: you can have a taste disorder even though your sense of smell is perfectly normal.

Common Causes of Taste Disorders

As with smell disorders, the most common cause of taste disorders is normal aging. Other causes include:

▶ Medications
▶ Neurologic disorders
▶ Common medical conditions
▶ Taste impairment after ear, nose, and throat surgery

Normal Aging

Taste decline due to aging is much less common and severe than the decline in your sense of smell due to aging. Nonetheless, your ability to identify the basic tastes (sweet, salty, bitter, sour, and **umami**, a relatively new category that includes savory tastes) decreases as you age. By the time you are 65 and older, sweet and salty are the most difficult tastes to recognize in your food. As such, older people tend to oversalt and oversweeten their food.

> **Taste declines much less due to aging than does the sense of smell.**

Medications

Medications are one of the most common causes of taste loss. Caroline, the patient mentioned in Chapter 1, who lost much of her sense of smell and taste while on a combination of medications for migraines and mild hypertension, is just one of many people whose ability to taste is impaired by medication.

Although taste alteration is a known side effect of many common medications, we still don't know as much as we should about these taste-alteration side effects since very little research has been done in this area. Most of what we know about these side effects is from case reports. For example, in the elderly, medication is reported to cause taste alteration in 10 to 30 percent of patients. (Medications can also cause an unpleasant taste simply by dissolving in the mouth or being chewed—a common example is aspirin—but this is not a long-lasting effect on taste or taste perception.)

> **Prescribed medications are one of the most common causes of altered taste.**

Medications can alter taste perception by:

▶ Reducing the quality and production of saliva
▶ Interfering with the taste buds and their taste cells
▶ Causing inflammation of the cells lining the mouth, tongue, and pharynx
▶ Altering the nerves and brain function involved in the taste system

Several common medications can reduce saliva production:

▶ Antidepressants, such as amitriptyline (Elavil) and paroxetine (Paxil)

Umami A relatively new term for one of the five basic tastes, roughly meaning "savory" or "meaty." (The other four basic tastes are sweet, sour, bitter, and salty.)

▶ Antihistamines, such as diphenhydramine (Benadryl)
▶ Diuretics, such as furosemide (Lasix)
▶ Anticholinergics, such as tolterodine (Detrol)

Most of these medications cause dry mouth by blocking a **neuro-transmitter** (a chemical that relays signals between nerves and the brain) called **acetylcholine**, which is also necessary for salivary glands to release saliva into the mouth.

Several medications used to control high blood pressure and heart failure interfere with the action of zinc in the salivary glands and taste cells. Zinc action is necessary for saliva to digest our food and for taste cells to function normally. Captopril (Capoten) and Lisinopril (Prinivil) are examples of these medications. Taste alteration occurs in about one out of ten people who use these medications.

Some medications can impair the function and renewal of taste buds and taste cells. Chemotherapy, for example, can interfere with the body's normal, routine replacement of taste cells.

Medications used in the treatment of Parkinson's disease, like levodopa, and antiseizure medications, like phenytoin (Dilantin) and carbamazepine (Tegretol), interfere with taste cells and the nerve pathways of the taste system. Another example is topiramate (Topamax), commonly used for migraine headaches and seizures. It can affect taste generally, and it is particularly known to affect the taste of carbonated beverages, causing them to taste flat or metallic. Cholesterol-lowering medications such as atorvastatin (Lipitor) and pravastatin (Pravachol) can cause taste alteration in a small number of cases. The exact mechanism for the alterations is unknown.

Radiation Therapy

Radiation therapy for head and neck cancers can severely impair taste. It damages the salivary glands, causing loss of saliva production. It can lead to mouth infections, facial nerve damage, and direct injury to the taste

---

Neurotransmitter A chemical that relays information from one nerve cell to another.
Acetylcholine One of a number of chemicals called neurotransmitters that relay signals in the brain and the junction between a nerve and muscle. Acetylcholine plays a role in a number of the body's physical responses, including stimulation of the salivary gland to release saliva. It also stimulates muscles to contract when we want them to move.

Medications Associated with Taste Disturbance

Category of Medication	Example of Medication
Anti-inflammatory	Allopurinol
Nonsteroid anti-inflammatory	Ibuprofen
Antibiotic	Tetracycline
	Penicillin
Anticholinergic	Tricyclic antidepressants (e.g., amitriptyline [Elavil, Endep])
	Trihexyphenidyl (Artane)
	Benztropine (Cogentin)
Antidepressants	Lithium carbonate
	Amitriptyline (Elavil, Endep)
	Paroxetine (Paxil)
Calcium channel blockers	Nifedipine
	Diltiazem (Cardizem)
Carbonic anhydrase inhibitors	Acetazolamide (Diamox)
Cardiac arrhythmia drugs	Propranolol
	Amiodarone
Cancer drugs	Methotrexate
	Vincristine
Cholesterol drugs	Atorvastatin (Lipitor)
	Pravastatin (Pravachol)
Diuretics	Hydrochlorothiazide
	Furosemide
Hypoglycemic drugs (oral)	Phenformin
	Glipizide
Parkinson's disease drugs	Levodopa
	Selegiline (Eldepryl, Zelapar)
Seizure drugs	Topiramate (Topamax)
	Diphenylhydantoin (Dilantin)
	Carbamazepine (Tegretol)

buds and their cells. Because taste buds and their taste receptors are capable of regenerating, taste usually recovers within a year after radiation therapy. Dryness of the mouth, however, can persist because scarring of the salivary gland may be permanent. Many available preparations of artificial saliva are available to help this condition and improve taste.

Smoking

Frequent smoking can also result in mild taste loss, due primarily to chemicals in the cigarette itself and in the smoke. When you stop smoking, your sense of smell and taste usually improves. However, recovery could take as long as the length of time you smoked.

> **Taste alteration from a neurologic disorder is usually very mild.**

Neurologic Disorders

Some neurologic disorders directly affect the taste system. They can cause partial or total loss of taste, or unpleasant tastes. It is very important for physicians and family members to recognize that these neurologic disorders can be associated with altered taste and enjoyment of food because unrecognized—and hence untreated—these impairments can lead to decreased appetite and weight loss in people whose health may already be fragile.

Often, multiple factors contribute to taste loss in patients with brain disorders. These include the part of the brain affected, the medications used, as well as other medical conditions, such as diabetes.

One disorder that can be associated with taste loss is **Bell's palsy**, which causes muscle weakness or paralysis on one side of the face. Bell's palsy impairs one's ability to smile or close an eye. Most of the time the exact cause of Bell's palsy is unknown, but we do know that it brings about inflammation of the facial nerve, which is adjacent to another nerve, the **chorda tympani**, that passes the sense of taste from the tongue (Figure 3). The chorda tympani can also be inflamed in

---

Bell's palsy A neurologic disorder that causes inflammation of the facial nerve (seventh cranial nerve). It causes partial or total paralysis of the facial muscles on one side of the face and alters basic taste (sweet, sour, bitter, salty, and umami) on the same side of the tongue as the facial paralysis.

Chorda tympani The nerve that joins the fifth nerve to the seventh nerve and carries basic taste information from the front two-thirds of the tongue.

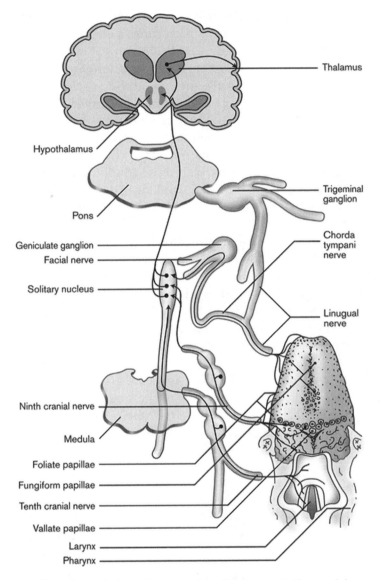

Figure 3 View of the whole taste system from the tongue to the cranial nerves 5, 7, 9, and 10 to the nerve pathways of the brain.

the case of Bell's palsy, leading to loss of taste on one side of the tongue. Four out of five people with Bell's palsy make a complete recovery.

Taste problems from disorders that damage the brainstem or brain, such as strokes, brain tumors, or multiple sclerosis (MS), are very uncommon, and patients with these conditions seldom notice or mention them. This might be because other symptoms, such as weakness or double vision, are so much more distressing. One study of people with taste disorders from strokes and MS showed areas of brain injury on MRI scans in the regions of the brain important for taste recognition. When people with these conditions do report taste problems, the symptom is usually mild and felt only on one side of the tongue. In very rare cases, taste problems can be the first symptom in MS.

Alzheimer's disease frequently affects the smell system. It rarely affects the taste system alone. Patients can also develop loss of appetite, weight loss, and depression.

People with seizure disorders sometimes experience an abnormal smell or taste very briefly, usually for less than two minutes, at the onset of the seizure. This sensory event is called an aura. Taste auras also occur but are rare compared to smell auras. Taste auras are frequently very unpleasant and are described as the taste of rotten apples, stale cigarettes, or vomit. Smell and taste auras are associated with seizure activity that begins in specific areas of the brain (the surface of the brain or the inner surface of the temporal lobe) (Figure 4). Medications used to control seizures, such as phenytoin (Dilantin) or levetiracetam (Keppra), can reduce or stop these auras.

Migraine

People with migraine are occasionally sensitive to different tastes but are more likely to report heightened sensitivity to odors. Less than 1 percent of people with migraine experience unpleasant smell as part of the migraine attack. (See also the migraine section in Chapter 1.)

Other Medical Conditions

Half of all people with low thyroid function and normal smell develop taste symptoms. The ability to taste all five primary tastes (salty, sweet, bitter, sour, and umami) is impaired, with the bitter taste being the most affected. Taste usually returns to normal with thyroid hormone supplementation.

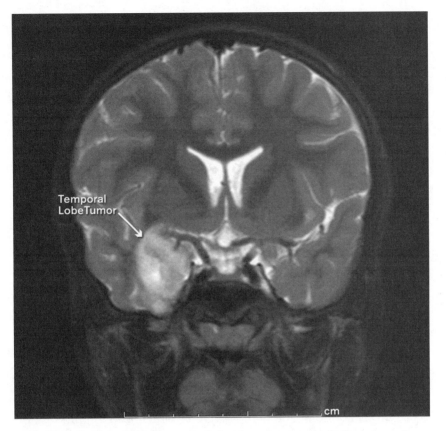

Figure 4   MRI of the brain (front view) showing a large tumor in the temporal lobe causing a seizure and preceded by a smell aura.
Image courtesy David Leake, MD, Austin Radiology Associates, Austin, Texas.

People with liver and kidney disorders commonly have taste symptoms. They are less able to detect any of the five basic taste categories. Unpleasant taste (dysgeusia) frequently occurs. This often leads to poor appetite and weight loss. Causes of taste impairment in liver and kidney disorders include:

► Reduced saliva production
► Low zinc levels
► Impaired function of the taste receptors
► Some medications used in treatment of these conditions

In these conditions, taste usually improves when liver and kidney functions improve; it often also improves with dialysis in kidney disease. Eliminating or changing some offending medications and adding zinc and vitamin therapy can also be helpful.

People with diabetes, like Genevieve, can often develop a taste disorder, as diabetes reduces sensitivity to the five basic tastes for reasons such as:

▶ Medications used to control the disease
▶ Reduced saliva production
▶ Damage to the nerves that control taste

Good control of diabetes can often lead to taste improvement.

Gastroesophageal reflux disease (GERD), also known as heartburn or acid indigestion, is a fairly common problem but not always recognized as a possible cause of taste alteration. This condition can lead to a chronic cough and altered taste due to irritation and inflammation of the lining of the mouth and tongue. In GERD, stomach acid escapes from the stomach into the esophagus and the throat. The stomach acid is very irritating and has a terrible taste.

Other chemicals besides gastric acid can cause taste alteration. One patient lost all her taste in a restaurant after taking a gulp of water from a glass that mistakenly contained bleach. She damaged the inside of her mouth and tongue, probably destroying most of the taste cells and receptors. She had very little taste improvement one year later. Excessive temperature, bacteria, and viral infections cause inflammation of the mouth and tongue and can, thereby, cause taste changes. An example of this is poor oral and dental hygiene, which lead to gum disease and tooth decay. These taste changes are usually temporary and disappear when the inflammation clears up.

Sjögren's syndrome mostly affects women in their thirties and forties and is frequently a cause of taste impairment. In Sjögren's disease, the body produces abnormal antibodies that attack different parts of the

---

Gastroesophageal reflux disease (GERD) A common medical condition caused by gastric acid spilling out of the stomach and traveling up the esophagus into the mouth and throat. GERD causes heartburn and can also cause a bad taste in the mouth. When left untreated, GERD can cause many other medical complications, including esophageal ulcers, chronic pulmonary disease, and Barrett's esophagus (a change in the lining of the esophagus that increases the risk of developing esophageal cancer).

Sjögren's syndrome A chronic autoimmune condition in which the white blood cells attack the glands that produce saliva. This condition affects as many as 4 million Americans.

body, particularly the salivary glands, the lining of the mouth and tongue, the cranial nerves, and nerves of the extremities. Taste often improves with treatment, which includes steroids, chemotherapy, and the use of artificial saliva.

Taste Impairment after Ear, Nose, or Throat Surgery

An important nerve that carries taste information from the front two-thirds of the tongue, known as the chorda tympani (shown in Figure 3), is located in the middle ear. On occasion it can be stretched or bruised during middle ear surgery, which can lead to taste alteration on one side of the tongue.

When taste is impaired, medical disorders such as low thyroid, liver and kidney disorders and GERD should be ruled out.

The disturbance is generally brief, and patients usually recover completely. Because taste function is still normal in the palate, the pharynx, and the other side of the tongue, these normal areas tend to minimize symptoms from the impaired side.

Tonsil surgery can injure the ninth cranial nerve, which supplies taste to the back one-third of the tongue. Occasionally taste symptoms occur after this surgery, but, again, it is quite uncommon—less than 1 percent of cases—and short-lived. In one large study of 3,500 cases, only 11 patients (0.3%) reported taste problems, all of whom recovered in a few months.[1]

People with obstructive sleep apnea, which is associated with frequent snoring and excessive daytime sleepiness, may have surgery to the very back part of the palate to correct this problem. Studies have found that as many as 10 percent of patients may develop taste problems after this surgery. The reason for taste alterations in these cases appears to be the lessened ability of food odor molecules and air to pass to the back of the **nasopharynx** (the uppermost part of the throat) to reach the smell organ.[2] This situation results in loss of flavors, which patients perceive as a loss of taste.

Nasopharynx The connection between the nose and the region behind the tongue and upper throat. Food molecules in the mouth reach the olfactory organ in the nose through this pathway

People who have surgery for cancer of the larynx (voice box) often have taste problems, for the same reason as in palate surgery for snoring. The larynx surgery interferes with the normal pathway through which air and food molecules reach the smell organ through the back of the throat. This damage leads to loss of flavors, which is interpreted as taste loss.

During general anesthesia or in emergency breathing conditions, a breathing tube is inserted through the nose or mouth and into the throat to access the airway. Once in a while the **lingual nerve**, which runs along the base of the tongue, is very mildly injured by the laryngoscope, an instrument that moves the tongue away so a breathing tube can be inserted down the back of the throat into the airway. This can lead to mild taste impairment on the injured side of the tongue. It usually recovers without long-term effects.

Taste changes, such as taste loss and unpleasant taste, can occur with some dental procedures, as well. Dentures and dental apparatus can be culprits. This is infrequent, and only isolated case reports have been documented. The taste change is possibly due to an allergy to the dental material.

References

1. Tomita H, Ohtuka K. Taste disturbance after tonsillectomy. *Acta Otolaryngologica Supplement* 2002;546:164–172.

This article discusses in detail the uncommon short-term taste symptoms a person may develop after tonsil surgery.

2. Badia L, et al. The effect of laser assisted uvulopalatoplasty on the sense of smell and taste. *Rhinology* 2001;39:103–106.

This study discusses palate surgery, which is commonly performed in people with sleep apnea, a condition causing nighttime snoring that reduces the amount of room oxygen that gets to the lungs and brain and leads to excessive daytime sleepiness. Palate surgery can impair taste is some people, as described in the article.

Lingual nerve A branch of the trigeminal (fifth) nerve that runs along the base of the tongue. It receives basic taste, temperature, texture, and spiciness information from the front two-thirds of the tongue. The taste sensation nerve fibers enter the chorda tympani nerve on route to the facial (seventh cranial) nerve.

3

Temperature, Texture, and Spice: How Does the Smell and Taste System Work?

In this chapter, you will learn:

▶ How the smell and taste systems are structured
▶ How smell and memory are related
▶ What happens when we smell and taste
▶ Some history of smell and taste

To understand what's gone wrong when you have a smell or taste disorder, it helps to understand how we smell and taste in the first place. Our senses of smell and taste are separate in some ways, but they are also closely interrelated. Having an impaired sense of smell without it also affecting one's sense of taste is uncommon.

How We Smell

What is the organ that senses smell? You probably answered "the nose," as most people would. But in fact, the organ that senses smell lies *within* the nose—up in the highest part of the nose, to be precise—within the **mucous membrane**, the moist outer layer of the lining inside the nose, which is the first structure to come into contact with the air and odor molecules we breathe. The smell organ is made up of the **olfactory cells**, which are actually nerve cells that function as receptors for the sense of smell. There are about 6 million of these specialized cells in each human nostril—many more in some animals, who have much better smell capabilities. (Your family dog has about 4 billion specialized nerve cells within his smell organ.)

Each olfactory cell has numerous small, thin, hairlike structures called cilia (see Figure 1, page 5), which are bathed in mucus and are stimulated by odor molecules when they enter the nose. Attached to the cilia are olfactory receptors, the part of the smell organ that actually makes contact with the odor molecules.

We are still learning about these olfactory receptors. Scientists Richard Axel and Linda Buck earned the Nobel Prize in 2004 for their work on olfactory receptors. They discovered that hundreds of different types of olfactory receptors are organized in families and subfamilies, which helps to explain how we use our sense of smell to recognize so many different odors and flavors.

Once the olfactory cells have grabbed onto the odor molecules, they send that information to the brain via a long thin nerve fiber called an **axon**. Many axons from many olfactory nerve cells run together and pass inside of the skull by way of the cribriform plate to form the **olfactory nerve** (see Figure 5).

Mucous membrane Linings for many body cavities—such as the nostrils—that contain lubricants and secretions. The nasal mucous membranes allow odors to dissolve so that the olfactory receptors can detect them.

Olfactory cells Specialized nerve cells found within the smell organ, olfactory cells have an outer nerve process that is capped with cilia that contacts the nasal mucous membrane and an axon that forms the olfactory nerve on the way to the olfactory bulb.

Axon A long, slender projection of a nerve cell that conducts electrical impulses, sending signals to and from the brain. Cilia project from one end of the olfactory receptor cells, collecting odor information, while axons project from the other, transmitting this information to the brain.

Olfactory nerve A collection of axons from many olfactory cells that travel through the cribriform plate on their way to the olfactory bulb.

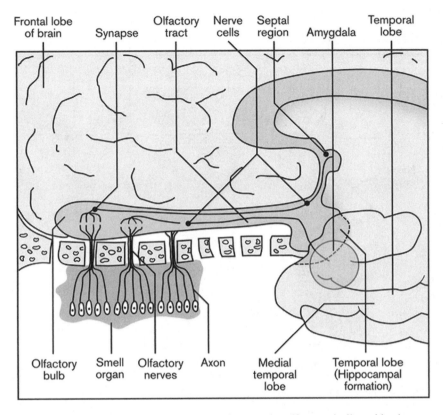

Figure 5   The smell organ and its connections to the olfactory bulb and brain.

The olfactory nerve continues on to the olfactory bulb (Figure 5) to contact other nerve cells. The axons from these nerve cells leave the olfactory bulb to form the **olfactory tract** (Figure 6).

Actually, each person has two olfactory bulbs and tracts—one for each nostril. Like other senses, such as sight and hearing, smell is processed on both sides of the brain. For example, odors that enter the left nostril stimulate the left side of the smell organ and the left olfactory bulb and nerves and then travel to both sides of the brain. (This partially explains why you can still smell some things when you have a cold that plugs up one nostril but not the other, although your smell may be somewhat impaired. More about this phenomenon is explained in the section on how your sense of taste works.)

Olfactory tract A narrow tract of white nerve fibers that extends from the olfactory bulb into various parts of the brain.

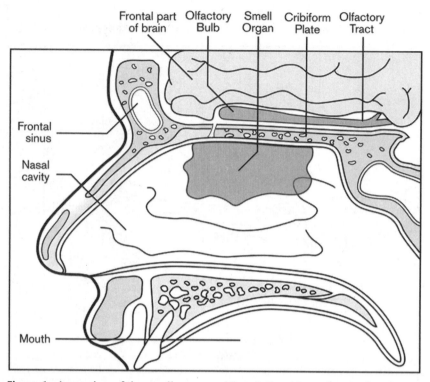

Figure 6   Inner view of the smell organ and its relationship to the nasal cavity and brain.

The olfactory tract continues on the undersurface of the brain to branch in many different directions, including to areas of the brain that are involved in memory and emotion.

All of these areas of the brain are important to our smell and taste system and to the way our sense of smell is experienced. For example, when you smell apple pie you might experience pleasant memories of your grandmother or holidays with the family. Or when you smell certain flowers, you might be reminded of your wedding day. The strong emotional feelings associated with the smell system are generally more pronounced than those with senses such as hearing and sight.

So how does the smell organ, in its place within the nose, receive odors to send on to the brain? First, from the air we breathe—although only 10 percent of the air we inhale reaches the smell organ.

Sniffing plays a key role in odor detection. It can be voluntary, such as when we take a sniff to smell something, but it usually occurs involuntarily and is part of the normal smell mechanism. When we sniff, we draw in more air—with its accompanying odor molecules—and the odor remains in contact with the smell organ longer.

The smell organ also receives odors and flavors from food when it is in our mouths. This is very important because it is how we identify, appreciate, and enjoy our food. The odors and flavors of our food reach the smell organ through the back of the throat as we swallow and exhale. When aromas and flavors contact the nerve cells in the smell organ, an electrical impulse is triggered. The impulse travels through the nerve pathways with information about the odor and flavor of the food. Our smell system is very important in our acceptance and pleasure of food. It is responsible for the pleasant feelings that accompany an enjoyable dinner.

> **The smell organ in the upper nose is made up of many smell receptors and their nerve processes.**

How We Remember Odors

You may have noticed that the smell of a gardenia perfume that your mother wore when you were small suddenly catapults you back to your childhood home, watching her get ready to go out to dinner. Or the scent of chalk and pencil erasers may conjure a vivid mental picture of your fifth-grade classroom, with its scuffed floor and scratched-up desks. A whiff of suntan oil may transport you to the beach almost as completely as a flight to Aruba.

Odors can be the best cues to memories. Memories that are triggered by odors are more emotional and more vivid than memories triggered by sights or sounds. (Despite their power, however, studies show that odor-triggered memories are no more accurate than memories triggered by any of the other senses.)

Why do odor memories result in particularly strong emotional responses? One possibility is that the nerve pathways of the smell system travel through regions of the brain central to emotional responses. Together, these areas are called the **limbic system**. Other sensory systems,

---

Limbic system A complex set of brain structures that includes the hypothalamus, the hippocampus, and the amygdala. The limbic system controls many basic functions of the body involving emotion and motivation, including experiencing pleasure.

> The main functions of the smell system are to identify odors in the environment and to help recognize flavors in our food.

such as sight and hearing, have fewer connections to the limbic system. This may explain why odors often cause stronger emotional responses than sights or sounds. Another theory is that odors may have a stronger emotional component since we rarely experience certain odors. Therefore, the brain is more likely to remember something good or bad associated with a particular odor when you first smelled it.

Our ability to detect an odor is generally good, but our ability to correctly identify the odor is much less accurate. Odors that are familiar are much easier to remember than new odors. Interestingly, women recognize and identify odors much better than men. As we age, the sense of smell weakens in both men and women. However, smell tends to decline much earlier in men than in women.

How We Taste

Three systems are actually involved in taste: the sensory (trigeminal), the smell, and the taste systems. The sensory, or trigeminal, system, which is shown in Figure 2 (see Chapter 1, page 9), tells the brain about the temperature, texture, and spiciness of food. The flavor of food depends on an intact smell system, as mentioned in the previous sections of this chapter. And the basic food tastes of sweet, sour, bitter, salty, and umami depend on an intact taste system.

So, for example, when you eat grilled barbecued beef with hot sauce, your **trigeminal system** tells you that the food is spicy, hot, and chewy, but the flavor and savory taste of the beef is identified by the smell and taste system working together. This is important to know because most

---

Trigeminal system The name given to the nerve system that includes the trigeminal nerve and its connections to the trigeminal nuclei in the brainstem, the thalamus, and the surface of the brain. This system provides information about pain, touch, and temperature of the face and inside of the mouth, and temperature, texture, and spice recognition of the food and drink we eat.

disorders of smell and taste do not affect the trigeminal system. If you have a smell and taste disorder, you still can enjoy your food by adding spices and changing its temperature and texture.

The sensory system of our mouth and nose is made up of the fifth cranial nerve, also called the **trigeminal nerve**, and its nerve pathways to the brain. (There are twelve pairs of cranial nerves—24 total—serving the sensory systems of the head and neck.) The trigeminal nerve carries pain, touch, and temperature sensations from the face, eyes, inside and outside of the mouth, and the tongue (see Figure 2, page 9). It also carries information about the texture, temperature, and spiciness of the food you eat. When your dentist numbs your mouth to do dental work, she is numbing some of the nerve fibers of the trigeminal nerve.

> The main function of the trigeminal system is to identify texture, temperature, and spiciness of food and pain and touch sensation in the mouth.

Nerve fibers that carry this sensory information connect to the **trigeminal nucleus** in the brainstem (see Figure 2, page 9). The trigeminal nerve also transmits basic taste information from the front two-thirds of the tongue through one of its branches called the lingual nerve (see Figure 1, page 5).

Our taste system, which mainly recognizes the five basic tastes of sweet, sour, bitter, salty, and umami (savory), is made up of numerous taste receptors that are located all over the surface of the tongue, on the roof of the mouth, in the back of the throat, and in the upper voice box region (larynx).

These taste receptors are located within structures called taste buds. Our taste system consists of about 10,000 taste buds, each containing 100 to 150 taste receptor cells. Each taste receptor cell has a nerve

---

Trigeminal nerve (fifth cranial nerve) The nerve responsible for sensation in the face and mouth. It also recognizes texture, temperature and spiciness of food.

Trigeminal nucleus The area *in the brainstem* where all sensory nerve fibers from the face *and mouth* end. All sensory information from the face, including touch, position, pain, and temperature, is carried to the trigeminal nucleus.

Our taste system consists of about 10,000 taste buds each containing 100 to 150 taste receptor cells.

process that sticks out on the surface of the taste bud. All these nerve processes from many taste cells are called **microvilli**. Their purpose is to contact food and drink molecules so we can taste them (Figure 7). You can see some of your taste buds on the back surface of your tongue—a row of small bumps that form a *V* shape. These bumps are called vallate papillae. The edge of the tongue from front to back has small bumps and an irregular surface that contains taste buds full of taste receptors called **foliate papillae**; the center and front of the tongue have little bumps and an irregular surface called **fungiform papillae** (Figure 8). The foliate and fungiform papillae are much more difficult to see with the naked eye.

It was once thought that taste receptors in different locations only recognized certain specific taste sensations; however, more recent research has shown that every taste receptor can recognize all taste sensations. There are some minor differences, though: the front two-thirds of the tongue recognizes sweet and salt the best while the back one-third of the tongue recognizes bitterness and umami (savory) the best.

Because taste receptors are so widespread, the taste system is less vulnerable than the smell system, which depends on one small smell organ in the nose. Therefore, disorders of basic taste are far less common. Still, cases do exist in which all the taste receptors can be impaired at one time. The best example is the use of medications that impair taste, as mentioned in Chapter 2. Since the medication gets into the bloodstream, it is carried to all the taste receptors; it can also affect saliva, which can impair the ability of a taste receptor to function properly. Another example of such widespread damage is exposure to a toxin—like the woman also mentioned in Chapter 2, who accidentally took a gulp from a glass containing bleach at a restaurant. The bleach

---

Microvilli Antenna-like structures that arise from all the taste receptors and are located in each taste bud. Microvilli contact the food molecules on the tongue so that their taste can be identified.

Foliate papillae Tiny bumps on the front and side edges of the tongue that contain taste buds. They are not well seen by the naked eye.

Fungiform papillae   Small bumps on the center and front of the tongue that contain taste buds. They are not well seen with the naked eye.

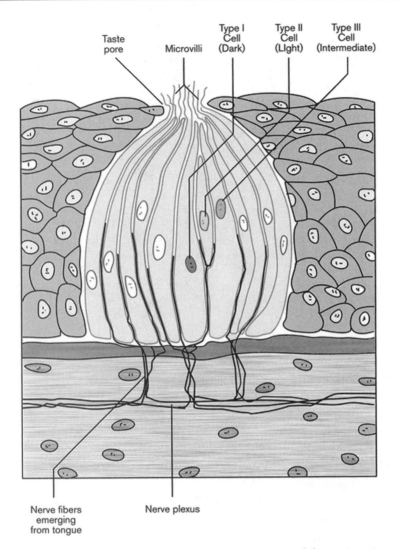

Figure 7   Enlarged view of a taste bud from the tongue containing many taste cells and nerve endings.

probably destroyed many of her taste receptors, and she may never completely regain her sense of taste.

One of the best terms to describe the way food stimulates the trigeminal system is the word *pungency*. Pungency can mean a fairly wide range of sensations, from warmth or irritation to severe pain. To describe a food's pungency, we tend to use terms such as *spicy, hot, cooling, burning, sharp, biting, tingling,* and *stinging*. Foods that

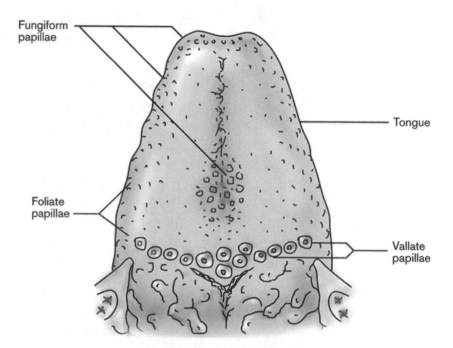

Figure 8   Top view of the tongue showing three different kinds and locations of taste papillae. Each is made up of numerous taste buds and taste cells.

The main function of the taste system is to recognize five taste sensations: sweet, sour, bitter, salty, and umami (savory).

strongly stimulate the trigeminal system are characteristic of non-Western cultures, including India, China, and Korea, as represented by dishes such as curries, Szechuan dishes, and kimchi. Adding Tabasco sauce, jalapeno peppers, or horseradish to many foods stimulates the trigeminal system.

The chemical substances in food that give us pungent flavors include capsaicin, a chemical found in chili that causes a burning, tingling, biting sensation, and menthol, which is found in peppermint oil and causes cooling, numbing, and burning sensations. Also, cuminaldehyde, found in cumin, results in burning, tingling, and numbing sensations.

The sensations of some of the trigeminal food stimulants are dependent on temperature. This is not a surprise because we have already mentioned that the trigeminal system is responsible for our appreciation of the temperature of food. When a very spicy sauce is added to warm or hot food, the spiciness of the sauce is increased and can lead to a burning sensation. When menthol is added to already cold food, the sensation of cooling and numb feeling of the menthol is increased.

Because taste receptors are so widespread in the mouth and back of the throat, taste loss is much less common than smell loss.

In general, studies suggest foods that stimulate the trigeminal system enhance our food experience; but it has also been suggested that overstimulation of the trigeminal system by chili or peppers can actually reduce taste and flavor of some foods, especially sweet ones.

The pungent sensations in our mouth and face, sensed by the trigeminal nerve, have a slow onset, which may last from 2 to 10 minutes depending on the strength. For example, if you've ever tasted an extra-spicy pepper or chili hot sauce (like those labeled "911" or "Call the fire department!"), you know that the burning sensation in your mouth can last for quite awhile. If you scoop up multiple mouthfuls of that hot sauce with your corn chips, it can further increase the intensity of the irritation.

This example contrasts with the way that flavors and **tastants** (substances that stimulate the sense of taste) are perceived. Flavors like vanilla and chocolate and general tastants like sweet, sour, bitter, and salty usually are most intense at the beginning and only last a few seconds.

In 1998, researchers Dr. Rob S. T. Linforth and Dr. Andrew J. Taylor developed a method to study how flavor is recognized during eating. They studied air that is exhaled from the nose during eating and found that a person recognizes the flavor intensity of a food at the same time that the food odor appears in the nose. The fact that our recognition of a flavor is simultaneous with the recognition of the odor further underscores how important our sense of smell is to our sense of taste.

Intensity and duration of flavor are dependent on the method of flavor release. Think of eating a banana as opposed to drinking a banana

---

Tastants Substances that stimulate the sense of taste. There are five major tastants: sweet, sour, salty, bitter, and umami (savory).

milkshake. When you first take a bite of an actual banana, you will appreciate the fruit flavor of the banana intensely and for a few minutes. But if, instead, you get the taste of banana from sipping a banana milk shake, you won't experience the banana flavor as intensely or for longer than 30 seconds. The reason: the appreciation of banana flavor rapidly disappears when the sweetness of the milk shake dissolves in the saliva and is swallowed.

Is it possible to have moderate to severe loss of smell and still have full appreciation of flavors? The answer is yes, but this does not happen very often. Doctors who treat people with smell and taste disorders have reported such cases. A study of 13 patients with this unusual combination of loss of smell but retained appreciation of flavors was conducted in 2005.[1] The study showed that the patients had abnormal scores on a standard smell test. However, when these flavors were placed on the middle of the tongue and the patients were told to block their noses, they were able to correctly identify the flavors. This response suggests that different parts of the smell organ may be stimulated, depending on where the odor is introduced. The front of the smell organ appears to sense odors passing through the nose while the back of the smell organ may sense odors coming from inside the mouth. This may explain why some people with viral infections and head injuries are still able to recognize odors and flavors even when they have significant smell loss.

People who can still perceive odors and flavors even when their ability to smell is impaired tend to be much less distressed, have a better appetite, and experience less depression because their ability to detect flavors is normal. I'm one of those lucky individuals, as have been a dozen or more of my patients. Although I lost 30 to 40 percent of my smell following a viral infection, my ability to identify flavors was not impaired.

Smell and Taste Throughout History

Smell and taste have been important to human beings throughout recorded history. In the ancient civilizations like Greece, Rome, and the Far East, spices and perfumes were used frequently in oils to care for the skin exposed to the hot and dry climate. These spices and perfumes were also used in some religious ceremonies.

The Romans believed that burning certain substances like sulfur or asphalt caused illnesses, including epilepsy. They also believed perfumes and spices had some medicinal properties. This concept was not really that far-fetched—it has been shown that essential oils can kill certain fungi, and certain Indian grasses are helpful in alleviating food poisoning.

Perfumes and spices were little known in Europe until the late Middle Ages and Renaissance era. In Europe, France became the leader in perfume development because of its very large flower industry. Louis XV, who reigned from 1715 to 1774, used perfumes extensively in his court. During conservative Victorian times in the late-eighteenth century, however, England passed a law that banned the use of perfumes and spices by women to attract men. (Interestingly, today some communities are seeking bans on perfumes and other strong body scents again, this time because of complaints that strong aromas give coworkers and others nearby headaches or nausea.)

It was also common thinking, dating back to early Roman times, that certain odors and tastes caused disease. This was especially true during the Black Death (bubonic plague) in the thirteenth and fourteenth centuries. In Western Europe in the eighteenth century, where the sewage systems were primitive, many people believed that the stench of sewage caused disease. (Of course, it was not the stench itself but the bacteria and other contaminants found in the sewage that bred illness.)

By the beginning of the nineteenth century, perfumes and spices played a major role in society, particularly in masking the more disagreeable everyday smells in the environment.

It was also known in the ancient world that perfumes and spice had medicinal properties and could ward off insects and bacteria. They were later shown to also control infections caused by Staphylococcus bacteria and various forms of tuberculosis bacteria.

Interestingly, before modern studies found that perfumes can kill bacteria and tuberculosis organisms, perfume workers in France in the late-nineteenth century appeared to have less incidence of tuberculosis and cholera compared to workers in other professions and in the population as a whole. This observation in the perfume industry helped to spur modern research into this subject.

Smell and taste loss, too, date back thousands of years. Smell loss was recognized in the earlier writings of Greece and Rome. Galen, a famous physician from 130 to 200 AD, described cases of smell loss. It was the theory at the time that smell loss was due to blockage of the small passages in the cribriform plate through which the olfactory nerves travel. In those days, the smell organ was incorrectly believed to be located in the center of the brain in cavities called ventricles that were filled with cerebral **spinal fluid**.

Causes of smell and taste impairment began to be recognized by physicians in the late-eighteenth and early-nineteenth century. Prior to the eighteenth century, physicians believed that if you could smell ammonia, your smell system was normal. But when physicians looking into smell and taste tested a patient known to have total smell loss and found that he had no trouble recognizing ammonia, they realized that a source other than the smell system had to be responsible for perceiving the pungent "odor" of ammonia. That source was the sensory system of the nose (trigeminal system). Many prominent neurologists who published textbooks in the early nineteenth century appeared to understand the basic anatomy and function of the smell and taste system; by this time they were especially aware that flavor recognition depended on an intact smell and taste system, and that the fifth (trigeminal) nerve was important in recognizing pungent odors such as ammonia.

At the time, the most common neurologic disorder known to be accompanied by altered smell and taste were seizures stemming from the temporal lobe and the **subfrontal region** of the brain due to head trauma or tumor. Smell and taste alterations were also recognized in upper respiratory viral infections and nasal obstructions such as **polyps** and tumors. Polyps are outgrowths of the lining of the inner nose that often develop in the presence of recurrent infection and swelling in the nasal passage. Polyps can be large or small. Many can become large enough to cause nasal blockage and interfere with air flow through the nose.

Due to major advances in all fields of science, the twentieth century was the most prolific so far in the field of smell and taste function and dysfunction. These advances included standardized smell testing, improved taste testing, and major developments in **computed tomographic (CT) scanning** and magnetic resonance imaging (MRI). In addition, there have been major advances in understanding the genetic makeup and function of the smell and taste receptors.

Spinal fluid Also known as cerebrospinal fluid or CSF, this protective fluid circulates around the brain and spinal cord and acts like a cushion, protecting the spine and brain from injury and supplies nutrients to the brain.

Subfrontal region The bottom part of the frontal lobe closest to the bony base of the skull.

Polyps Abnormal growths of tissue projecting from a mucous membrane.

Computed tomographic (CT) scanning A method of examining organs in the body by scanning them with x-rays and then using a computer to construct a series of three-dimensional cross-section images.

Reference

1. Landis BN, Frasnelli J, Reden J, et al. Differences between orthonasal and retronasal olfactory functions in patients with loss of sense of smell. *Archives Otolaryngology–Head and Neck Surgery* 2005;131(11):977–981.

This excellent article describes in detail how our smell system can identify smell—and even more importantly—flavor. It also explains how some people with severe smell loss can still retain the ability to identify food flavors.

4

Sniffing Out What's Wrong: How Smell and Taste Disorders Are Diagnosed

In this chapter, you will learn:

► What kinds of specialists diagnose smell and taste disorders
► What to expect when going to a specialist
► What tests are available to diagnose smell and taste disorders

Which Doctor to See? Seeking Medical Help

When Andrew, the truck driver from Chapter 1, experienced a loss of smell and taste after being rear-ended, he first went to see an ear, nose, and throat (ENT) specialist. So did Grace, the woman who found her smell and taste impaired after a stubborn cold. In fact, most of the causes of smell and taste disorders are within the specialties of ENT or neurology, which is the study of the brain and nervous system.

Viral infections of the upper nasal airway, sinusitis, nasal polyps, and disorders of the mouth and throat, including the tongue and inside of the palate, are generally diagnosed and treated by the ENT physician. Disorders of the olfactory nerve, olfactory bulb, and brain structures (frontal and **medial temporal lobes**)—such as brain tumors, seizures, stroke, head trauma, and **aneurysms** (a weakened, bulging area in one of the arteries that supplies blood to the brain)—are generally diagnosed and treated by the clinical neurologist. Neurologists also treat patients with Alzheimer's disease, Parkinson's disease, and multiple sclerosis, all of which frequently involve smell and taste impairments. You may have to see both types of specialists to determine the cause of your smell and taste disorder.

When you see the specialist, you will be asked many questions about your symptoms. These may include:

▶ Did you develop a change in your smell and taste after a cold or head injury?

▶ Did you start a new medication during the past two or three months?

▶ Do you have diabetes?

▶ Do you have a thyroid condition?

▶ What are your drinking and smoking habits? (It is important to be truthful about drinking and smoking.)

The ENT physician will carefully examine your nose and the inside of your mouth, including the tongue, gums, and teeth. Your oral hygiene will be carefully examined. (Poor oral hygiene may lead to an impaired ability to taste.) The ENT physician will order a CT scan of your sinuses and nasal passages to see if you have sinusitis, nasal polyps, or a tumor. For example, it is now possible to see the bone structures where the tiny olfactory nerves travel to enter the brain; however, CT does not show nerves and brain tissue from the areas in the base of the brain very well. These structures are hidden by bone, which the CT scan cannot see through.

Your ENT physician will also perform a **nasal endoscopy**, an important test for most people who have problems with their sense of smell.

Medial temporal lobe An area of the brain necessary in the storage of personal memories, general knowledge and facts, and odor recognition.

Aneurysm A weakened, bulging area in an artery—in the context of this chapter, in one of the arteries that supplies blood to the brain. Some aneurysms put pressure on surrounding brain tissue. Others can rupture, flooding the brain with blood. Most aneurysms do not rupture, but those that do are life-threatening.

Nasal endoscopy Passing a slender telescope through the nostril to examine the nasal passages and sinuses.

In this procedure, the doctor inserts a special tube called an endoscope into the nose. This tube has a magnifying lens and a camera at its tip, allowing the entire nasal passage and nasal smell organ to be seen. With endoscopy, the ENT doctor can see nasal polyps, inflammation, or scar tissue from viral infections and trauma. The endoscopy tube can also take a small tissue sample for biopsy, if necessary. This is the primary way to examine nasal structures and the olfactory organ. It is a safe office procedure and is performed with local anesthesia.

If you initially see a neurologist or are referred to one by your ENT specialist, you will be asked a number of additional questions that are related to the nervous system. For example, the neurologist will ask if you have headaches, double vision, facial numbness, balance problems, or trouble with your memory. The answers to these questions will help determine whether you have a problem with the olfactory nerve or the structures inside the brain.

The neurologist will conduct a detailed neurologic examination that includes testing the important cranial nerves related to smell, taste, and sensory function of the mouth and tongue. Those nerves are the trigeminal nerve (fifth cranial nerve), the **facial nerve (seventh cranial nerve)**, the **glossopharyngeal nerve (ninth cranial nerve)**, and the **vagus nerve (tenth cranial nerve)** (see Figures 2 and 3 on pages 9 and 27, respectively). You may also need magnetic resonance imaging (MRI) of the brain and olfactory region. MRI shows detailed images of many structures involved in smell: olfactory nerves, olfactory bulb, base of the frontal lobe, and the medial temporal lobe. It may show an abnormality such as a cyst or aneurysm (although these are uncommon causes of smell and taste disorders).

Facial nerve (seventh cranial nerve) This nerve controls the muscles of facial expression. It also carries information about basic taste (sweet, sour, bitter, salty, and umami) from the front two-thirds of the tongue by way of the chorda tympani nerve.

Glossopharyngeal nerve (ninth cranial nerve) A nerve that carries basic taste information from the back of the tongue and throat. It is also responsible for secreting saliva, swallowing, and receiving sensory information (pain, temperature, and touch) from the back parts of the tongue and throat.

Vagus nerve (tenth cranial nerve) This nerve conveys sensory information about the state of the body's internal organs, such as the stomach, liver, and kidneys, to the brain. It also carries basic taste information from the back of the throat and larynx to the brain.

The neurologist will probably also order some blood tests, including those that test thyroid and vitamin B_{12} levels.

Visiting a Smell and Taste Clinic

Some patients, like Andrew, Grace, and Caroline from Chapter 1, are referred to one of the few smell and taste specialty clinics and research centers in the United States (see Appendix A). Generally, these clinics can offer more detailed smell and taste testing, more treatment options, and patient education. They will take an even more detailed history of symptoms and provide more thorough smell and taste testing. Currently, few neurologists and ENT specialists outside of smell and taste clinics conduct detailed smell and taste testing during their examinations, but with ongoing education in this expanding field, this will hopefully change.

Smell and taste clinics will review all of your previous medical records and tests results and determine what further tests, if any, need to be done. At the completion of the evaluation, you will be given an explanation of your condition and information about the prognosis for recovery of your smell or taste disorder. Whether you recover partially, completely, or not at all, you will be given treatment strategies. We'll discuss more about those treatment and lifestyle approaches in the next chapter, but here is a brief description of the advice and guidance you might receive. At some clinics you will be counseled about changes in food preparation and offered recipes to improve your eating enjoyment. Weight loss and decreased appetite are often associated with smell and taste disorders and will be addressed. However, some people actually gain weight because they keep eating to find something that tastes satisfying. If you are depressed because of your condition, the clinic's mental health professional may recommend counseling or medication. Finally, the clinic staff may be able to provide treatment options and coping strategies for problems with unpleasant smells and tastes (see also Chapter 6 and the Recipes section at the back of this book).

Most neurologists and ENT specialists can conduct the basic diagnostic testing necessary to evaluate someone with a smell and taste problem. They can provide information about the cause and long-term effects of the disorders and suggest treatments. If the cause and long-term outcome of the smell and taste disorder is unclear or troubling or symptoms such as increasing weight loss, decreased appetite, and depression are present, a referral to a specialized smell and taste disorders clinic may be advised.

Specialized Smell Testing

For many years, physicians evaluated their patients' ability to smell by using small samples of coffee and wintergreen. In fact, many doctors still use this brief and incomplete smell assessment, although more comprehensive standardized smell tests are now available.

The most common and most reliable smell tests are the University of Pennsylvania Smell Identification Test (UPSIT) and the Brief Smell Identification Test (B-SIT). Both tests use a scratch-and-sniff format. These tests are very accurate and can determine how much an individual's smell is impaired. At a smell and taste specialty center, patients also typically undergo detailed taste testing using the whole mouth taste threshold test or the taste strip test (which are explained in greater detail in the Specialized Taste Testing section of this chapter).

The UPSIT was developed by Dr. Richard Doty, a prominent researcher and clinician who directs the Taste and Smell Center at the University of Pennsylvania, and his colleagues after they had spent many years studying smell in thousands of healthy men and women of various ages. This test has been available for more than 15 years and is very reliable.

The UPSIT includes four booklets, each containing 10 odors embedded in microcapsules on a strip at the bottom of each page. When the surface of the strip is scratched, the odor is released. The test is multiple choice, with four possible choices for each smell. After sniffing the strip, testers circle the response that they think best corresponds to the odor (see Figure 9). The UPSIT is not a timed test, and it is also available in many languages and designed to be culturally and ethnically sensitive. Forty odors are provided in the test, and each correct answer is given one point. A perfect score of 40 out of 40 is rarely achieved. An individual's total number of correct responses is compared to a table of normal responses, based on age and sex, to determine how well smell is functioning and how much smell has been lost.

Whether or not your score is considered "normal" depends on your age and sex, because as we age our sense of smell declines very

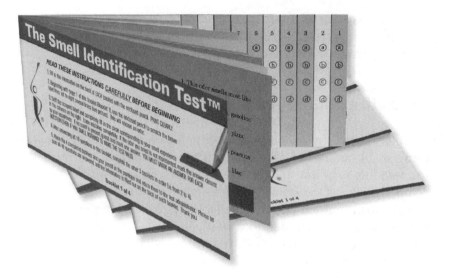

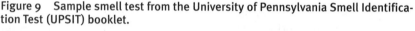

Figure 9   Sample smell test from the University of Pennsylvania Smell Identification Test (UPSIT) booklet.

Photograph courtesy of Sensonics, Inc., Haddon Heights, NJ.

gradually, and the male population overall does not smell as well as the female population. For example, a 40-year-old woman should score at least 38 out of 40 for her smell to be considered "normal" for her age and sex. For a 70-year-old woman, on the other hand, a score of 33 out of 40 is considered normal. Men of all ages will typically have lower normal UPSIT scores than women of the same age.

Andrew, the truck driver from Chapter 1, scored 14 out of 40, which represents severe smell loss. Grace, the woman who experienced smell and taste impairment after a cold, scored 16 out of 40, which is also severely impaired smell for her age and sex. On the other hand, Caroline, who had impaired smell after going on a combination of new medications for migraine and hypertension, scored 30 out of 40, which placed her in the mild to moderate smell loss category.

Another, shorter, version of the UPSIT is called the Brief Smell Identification Test, or B-SIT. The B-SIT, which contains only 12 different odors, can be given first. If it is abnormal, then the UPSIT can be used to confirm the initial abnormal results. A specialized version of the B-SIT is also available to screen for Alzheimer's disease, based on research suggesting that people with Alzheimer's disease are unable to identify 10 specific odors: menthol, clove, leather, strawberry, lilac, pineapple, smoke, soap, natural gas (mercaptan), and lemon. Although no special version of the smell test exists for Parkinson's disease, scientists have also discovered that people with Parkinson's disease have difficulty recognizing the following odors: licorice, coconut, banana, dill pickle, paint thinner, turpentine, cherry, and soap.

Another very brief smell test called the Quick Smell Identification Test (Q-SIT) has the same basic format as the UPSIT and B-SIT, except it only has three different odors to identify. It is helpful in diagnosing total smell loss in 65 percent of people, but it is not sensitive enough for everyone with smell loss, particularly those with mild smell impairment. It is useful for a quick evaluation at the bedside in hospital patients and some office patients who don't have any bothersome smell symptoms. However, for serious smell testing, the B-SIT and UPSIT are much more reliable and sensitive.

The Smell or Odor Threshold Test is a more specialized test unrelated to the UPSIT that provides further information about smell loss. Different concentrations of an odor are enclosed in multiple small tubes. The purpose of the test is to determine the lowest concentration of the odor that a person can smell. This test has also been standardized for the normal population as regards to age and sex. This test is usually done in specialized smell and taste centers.

Another standardized smell test that combines tests for odor identification, odor intensity, and odor threshold is called Sniffin' Sticks. This test is currently more widely available in Europe, where it was developed. It consists of multiple sets of pen-shaped odor dispensers, each set having the same odor at a different concentration. It is administered by another person and takes 30 minutes to complete. It is very reliable and provides detailed information about an individual's smell system.

The main purpose of the UPSIT, B-SIT, and other smell tests is to determine whether you have a smell disorder and, if so, to help understand its severity. These tests cannot determine the cause of the smell abnormality or whether it is coming from the smell organ or from damage to the nervous system.

Electrical Testing

The olfactory nerve cells generate electrical activity when odors pass through the nose. With the olfactory evoked potentials (OEP) test, electrodes placed on the scalp record these electrical signals, which travel from the olfactory nerve cells to the brain. This test is reliable and objective. It measures how well an individual's smell system is functioning. Disorders of the nerve pathways between the olfactory nerve and the brain can result in an abnormal or absent response. Both sides of the olfactory system can be compared using this test. It may be used to confirm impaired smell when a smell test is abnormal. However, the OEP test is not foolproof since one-third of patients may have an abnormal smell test but a normal OEP.

An abnormal smell test and an abnormal OEP strongly suggest impaired smell. The OEP can therefore be helpful in suspected medical-legal cases in which more objective testing is usually required. It may help identify mild impaired smell loss from head trauma following an accident that is of medical legal interest. Mild smell impairment with an abnormal OEP helps to reassure the legal system and physicians that the head injury was likely the immediate cause of the smell impairment. The OEP test is only available in smell and taste research centers because of the cost and limited use in most smell and taste problems.

Specialized Taste Testing

Taste testing is a bit more complicated and time-consuming than smell testing. It requires a person to administer the test as compared to the UPSIT, which is self-administered. One taste test, called the whole mouth taste test, uses sucrose (sweet), sodium chloride (salty), caffeine (bitter), and citrate (sour). Each one is mixed in low concentrations with distilled or bottled water. Before the test begins, individuals are told which tastes they will be trying to identify. The mixtures are then sipped, swished in the mouth, and spit out in order to try to identify each of the tastes. If tastes are not perceived or identifiable, higher concentrations of the taste solution are mixed and administered in the same way. This test can identify whether the taste sensation is absent or just less sensitive.

The whole mouth taste test will help to identify a primary taste problem or help confirm a smell disorder. Remember that primary taste disorders—that is, taste disorders without an accompanying smell problem—are fairly uncommon. In fact, the patients Grace and Caroline, both of whom reported that their food no longer tasted like it used to, scored normally on the whole mouth taste test, and Andrew only had mild impairments in tasting salty and sweet while bitter and sour were normal. But if they had been eating food with an accompanying aroma and a lot of flavor, they probably would have noticed that their meal tasted blander than expected because of the loss of flavor, or just sweet or tangy because their basic tastes were still mostly intact. This underscores just how much our sense of smell affects the way we taste.

Two tests are available to help with diagnosis when an individual suspects a taste problem on only one side of the tongue. One, developed in Germany, is called Taste Strips. It consists of paper strips with tastes of different concentrations embedded into them. These strips are placed on different parts of the tongue to see if tastes can be identified. The test has only been studied in people up to the age of 50, not in older people. Taste Strips can also be used for testing taste on the whole mouth and tongue. The advantage is that it does not require mixing any solutions. The other test, used in the United States, doesn't have a particular name. It consists of different solutions of the four basic tastes (sweet, sour, bitter, and salty), tested one at a time. Each solution is placed on one or both sides of the tongue using a pipette, which is similar to a large eyedropper. Each of the four solutions is administered separately to see if each taste can be identified, and whether it is stronger on one side or the other.

Summary of the Popular Smell and Taste Tests Available

Name of Test	How It Is Administered	What It Tells Us
Smell Tests		
1. University of Pennsylvania Smell Identification Test (UPSIT)	A 20-minute, self-administered test consisting of four booklets, each with 10 different scratch-and-sniff smells. Four answer options for each smell are given. Must choose one answer. Guessing is permitted.	How good a person's smell is compared to others of similar age and sex. Very reliable. Perfect score is 40/40.
2. Brief Smell Identification Test (B-SIT)	A 10-minute test consisting of one booklet of 12 different smells. Otherwise the same format as UPSIT.	Gauges a person's smell abilities compared to age only. This is a screening test; if the results are abnormal, the UPSIT should be given. Perfect score is 12/12.

(Continued)

Summary of the Popular Smell and Taste Tests Available *(Continued)*

Name of Test	How It Is Administered	What It Tells Us
3. Quick Smell Identification Test (Q-SIT)	A three-minute, self-administered test with only three odors. Otherwise the same format as the UPSIT and B-SIT.	A quick screening test for hospitalized patients, for testing larger groups, and for use when smell loss is suspected in someone without obvious symptoms. Score must be 3/3. If not, then the B-SIT or UPSIT should be done.
4. Odor Threshold Test	Odors of various concentrations are sniffed in multiple glass tubes.	How sensitive an individual's smell is. Determines the lowest concentration of an odor that a person can detect. The result is compared to known normal values for age and sex.
5. Sniffin' Sticks	An individual sniffs multiple sets of pen-like devices, each set with a different odor embedded at the top. Administered by a technician. Takes 45+ minutes to do. Mostly used in Europe.	Measures identification of odor as well as odor intensity and sensitivity in one test.
6. Olfactory Evoked Potentials (OEP)	Electrodes placed on the scalp record the response from the brain surface that occurs when an odor is delivered to the nose.	Tells whether the smell system is working normally. Unlike identifying odors, the OEP is not under a person's control.

Summary of the Popular Smell and Taste Tests Available *(Continued)*

Name of Test	How It Is Administered	What It Tells Us
Taste Tests		
1. Whole Mouth Test	Sweet, sour, bitter, and salty solutions are prepared each in small cups and in four different concentrations. A small amount of one solution is swished around inside the mouth. After 30 seconds it is spit out. The person tested has to identify the taste of each solution as sweet, sour, bitter, or salty. Takes 20–30 minutes.	Whether the taste receptors in the mouth for the basic tastes (sweet, sour, bitter, salty) are normal. A normal score is getting at least 50 percent of the taste solutions correct.
2. Taste Strips	Four different concentrations of basic tastes are embedded in filter paper strips. Each filter strip is placed in the mouth, then moved around the tongue and whole mouth. Individuals try to identify the taste (sweet, sour, bitter, salt). Takes 20–30 minutes. Developed in Europe but used in the United States. Does not require mixing (see 3 below).	Whether the taste system is normal or not and if a specific taste is impaired. A normal score is 9/16 or greater. Can also test different sides and parts of the tongue.
3. Pipette Solution Taste Test	Four solutions of each taste are made up. A small pipette, or thin tube, is used to draw up the taste solution. A small amount of solution is dropped from the pipette onto different parts of the tongue. Individuals must try to identify each taste. Takes over 30 minutes to administer.	Can measure taste in smaller areas of one or both sides of the tongue. Normal score is 50 percent or more correct.

What Does It Mean? Treatment Options and Lifestyle Changes

In this chapter, you will learn:

► How your smell and taste disorder may be treated
► Ways you can modify your cooking to improve your enjoyment of food
► Safety and hygiene precautions for living with smell and taste disorders

Some readers may be pleasantly surprised to see a chapter on treatment. For many years, doctors—and patients—believed that when the smell and taste systems were damaged, they were unlikely to recover. Few treatments were available. In the early part of the twenty-first century, research began to demonstrate that this thinking was wrong. It is now known that nerve cells and their connections can regenerate, and many people with smell and taste loss improve with time.

But even if you never fully recover your sense of smell, taste, or both, you can adapt your life in many ways so that you can still enjoy a delicious meal, appreciate the smell of spring flowers or a pleasant cologne, and avoid dangers posed by impaired smell or taste (such as gas leaks and spoiled food).

Education about Your Disorder

The first step toward treatment of any disorder is gaining understanding: knowing what your condition is, how it can be treated, and what happens next. After a thorough examination, including smell and taste testing, your specialist will put all the information from your history, examination, and diagnostic testing together to make a diagnosis and help you understand what you can expect. Will the condition improve, stay the same, or get worse? For example, smell and taste loss due to viral infections usually improves as the olfactory system heals. Smell and taste loss due to some medications will often improve or return to normal when the offending medication is stopped.

Treatment for Smell and Taste Disorders

Many of the causes of smell and taste impairment can be treated, and in some cases your sense of smell and taste will completely return to normal—either through successful treatment or simply with the passage of time. If your smell loss came on over a short period of time, you may be given a steroid nasal spray, especially if you have a cold or allergy. If you have a sinus infection, you may be treated with antibiotics. If your sinus infections are chronic or recurrent, you may need sinus surgery. These approaches often lead to improved smell and taste function.

Medications

The treatment for smell and taste loss caused by medications is simple and pretty obvious: changing the medications. Obviously, this solution is not always possible, and medication that has been prescribed by a doctor should never be discontinued or changed without first discussing it with him or her. But fortunately, many medications that cause smell and taste disturbances can be replaced with others that treat the same condition without causing these problems. Sometimes, just lowering the dose of a medication can help.

You may recall the story of Caroline from Chapter 1, who developed smell and taste loss after her doctor prescribed a combination of topiramate (Topamax) and diltiazem (Cardizem) to treat her migraine headaches and mild hypertension. When she returned to her doctors—she was seeing both a family physician and a neurologist—her neurologist first reduced the dose of topiramate she was taking, which partially improved the flatness Caroline tasted whenever she opened a fizzy soft drink. Her general smell and taste abilities were still impaired, however.

Ultimately, her family physician referred her to an ear, nose, and throat (ENT) physician, who referred her to a smell and taste clinic. When tested there, she scored 30 out of 40 on the University of Pennsylvania Smell Identification Test (UPSIT), which placed her in the mild to moderate smell loss category. Whole mouth taste testing was normal. Her treatment team told her that the cause of her continued smell and taste impairment was the combination of the two drugs, which are known to cause smell and taste loss. Fortunately, an alternative medication, propranolol (Inderal), which does not contribute to smell or taste loss, was available and could both lower her blood pressure and help with her migraines. In consultation with her family doctor and neurologist, Caroline slowly tapered off the other medications and switched to the new drug.

Over the next three months, Caroline's smell and taste both gradually returned to normal. (It can take as long as three to six months after medications are stopped for smell and taste to recover.) In the meantime, she learned to add flavorings to her food at two times the normal recommended amount, to use tiny amounts of **monosodium glutamate (MSG)** instead of extra salt, and to experiment with various spices she enjoyed.

Although MSG has gained a somewhat negative reputation as potentially causing health problems and negative reactions, research has largely discredited this. A 1995 report from the Federation of American Societies for Experimental Biology (FASEB) concluded that MSG was safe for most people when "eaten at customary levels." There was still a suggestion that some people might experience symptoms

---

Monosodium glutamate (MSG) A sodium salt that unlike regular salt has a very savory-taste similar to meat broth. It is representative of the newly accepted type of taste called *umami*. MSG is naturally present in many foods, such as tomatoes and beef. Twenty percent of the population cannot taste MSG due to a genetic defect. It is very safe and rarely causes nasal congestion, eye tearing, or migraine headaches. Much of the worry about using MSG is exaggerated. It has the same sodium content as regular salt but is available in a low-sodium form called Accent.

such as headache, numbness, weakness, and dizziness in reaction to MSG—something termed "Chinese restaurant syndrome"—but more recent research indicates that this connection is tenuous at best.[1]

After a Viral Infection

Smell and taste loss due to viral infections such as colds and sinusitis sometimes improves after the infection has fully gone away, but not always. Grace, the woman from Chapter 1 who could no longer enjoy her food or smell her shower gel after a severe cold, had been experiencing these symptoms for six months when she was referred to a smell and taste clinic—long after she'd stopped sniffling and sneezing.

Doctors told Grace that her smell function could continue to improve over the next 18 months or so, but that she might not make a full recovery. Over the next year, Grace's smell improved by about 50 percent. Her ability to recognize flavors also improved, but it was still impaired. But even though she did not recover her smell and taste functions completely, Grace has been able to enjoy her meals with strategies that the smell and taste clinic devised for her.

For example, Grace's favorite foods were bacon, eggs, and toast for breakfast, and roast beef and mashed potatoes for dinner. Her favorite condiments were ketchup, salsa, mustard, and vinegar. She kept eating these foods but learned to spice them up by adding salsa to her eggs and lemon pepper and garlic to her mashed potatoes. She also added tiny amounts of MSG to her roast beef and began preparing many of the special recipes found in Chapter 6 to heighten her appreciation of foods and flavors.

After an Accident

When Andrew, the truck driver who was rear-ended, went to see his ENT physician about his smell and taste symptoms, his physical examinations were normal, and no direct physiologic cause of his condition could be identified. The doctor gave him steroid nasal spray and told him his condition might improve with time. But after six months, little had changed for Andrew—his food still tasted bland, and there was no wake- up aroma with his morning coffee.

At a smell and taste clinic, UPSIT testing revealed that Andrew had severe smell loss, with a score of 14 out of 40, and mild impairment for salty and sweet in his whole mouth taste testing. This impairment was the result of the head injury he had sustained in his accident—a "whiplash" type of injury that caused his brain to rapidly shift forward and backward in the skull, putting strain on the olfactory nerves traveling through the base of the skull. Andrew also smoked two packs of cigarettes a day, which probably contributed to his smell and taste impairment and decreased sensitivity to salty and sweet tastes.

For most patients like Andrew, the damage to the smell and taste system done by a head injury cannot be repaired. During the 12 to 15 months following such an accident, smell and taste function may improve somewhat, but most of these patients likely will never recover completely. Andrew's doctors told him this, but they also told him that another factor was damaging his smell and taste that he *could* change: his smoking habit. Long-term smoking has been shown to impair smell and taste by up to 15 percent, and it can take many years to regain this loss after smoking stops. In Andrew's case, a 10 percent improvement could make a big difference in his condition because it is unlikely he will ever recover completely.

His treatment team urged Andrew to stop smoking and suggested he add various spices and condiments to his favorite foods—like salsa on his scrambled eggs and baked potatoes. He also began adding tiny amounts of MSG on the chicken and steak he loves to increase the savory taste, and he tried marinating chicken in fruit juices, spicy salad dressing, and sweet-and-sour sauce

Over the next 12 months, Andrew's smell and taste improved only slightly on testing. But he felt much better, particularly after he stopped smoking. Food tasted better to him, and he was able to maintain his weight and appetite. "Food tastes more alive," he said.

When Smell and Taste Problems Accompany Neurologic Disorders

Smell and taste alteration due to neurologic disorders such as multiple sclerosis and stroke usually improve with time and treatment of the disease process. On the other hand, smell and taste alterations in Alzheimer's disease, Parkinson's disease, and **dementia with Lewy bodies** usually continue to worsen and are not improved by medications used to treat these neurologic disorders. If you or a loved one has one of these disorders, the best way to improve the taste of food is by changing

---

Dementia with Lewy bodies A progressive brain disorder showing early features of visual hallucinations and memory loss and later development of impaired judgment and reasoning. Features similar to Parkinson's disease, such as stiffness, slow movement, and tremor, develop up to one year before to within one year of memory and cognitive decline.

food preparation—an approach that helped Mary, a 74-year-old woman with moderate Alzheimer's disease.

> Mary's daughter, who cared for her at home with the help of a caregiver who covered for her during her work hours, became worried when Mary began to lose weight and show less interest in her food. After consulting with Mary's physicians and trying a change of medication, her daughter brought her to a smell and taste clinic. Although Mary was unable to answer questions about any differences in the taste of food or the things that she smelled, her daughter recalled that her mother had mentioned in the past that food did not taste the same.
>
> Working with Mary's daughter, the treatment team compiled a list of Mary's favorite foods and provided food preparation tips that emphasized spices and flavor additives, as well as tiny amounts of MSG to increase the savory taste. They also explained to the daughter that her extended absences from home were probably a contributory factor, especially since the caregiver usually served Mary her meals and then went to clean up while Mary ate. People are very social, and we get some of our pleasure at meals from interacting with family and friends. The specialists suggested to Mary's daughter that she eat breakfast and dinner with her mother and that the sitter do the same at lunch.
>
> Mary soon began to regain her appetite and take in more calories. She put on three pounds in three weeks. Over the next three months she regained most of the weight she had lost.

Treating Dysosmia

Dysosmia—the perception of an abnormal, unpleasant smell—usually gets better on its own. It most commonly occurs following smell loss in head and nose injuries, viral infections of the nose and upper airway (colds), and chronic sinus infections—although it can be caused by any of the triggers of smell loss mentioned in Chapter 1. Dysosmia can be triggered by any environmental smell such as food, perfumes, or grass. It also can occur out of the blue without any trigger at all. If you experience dysosmia, be assured that it will eventually go away, even if the process is slow. The condition may take from three months to five years to resolve. For symptomatic relief in the meantime, there are several options.

NORMAL SALINE SOLUTION. Use a small syringe, usually measuring cubic centimeters (cc) and a small bottle of normal saline (salt solution), both of which can be purchased at any drugstore without a prescription. Fill the syringe with 10 cc of the normal saline solution, and then insert the filled syringe just past the entrance to one nostril and gently push the saline out of the syringe. Do this while seated, with your head down as far as possible. Stay in the head-down position for 20 seconds so the saline will reach the top of the nose. Then sit upright and let the over-flow saline drip out of your nose and wipe it off. Don't sniff or snort, or the saline will go into the back of the throat and escape the top of the nose. Repeat the process in the other nostril. Do this treatment three to four times per day.

A saline wash like this works by traveling to the top of the nose where the smell organ is located, temporarily blocking odors in the air from reaching the smell organ. One of the main reasons that dysosmia occurs is that when olfactory nerve cells are partially injured, the cells do not relay normal smell sensations. Instead, the person experiences an unpleasant, abnormal smell. Since many common environmental odors can trigger dysosmia, blocking these regular odors with normal saline prevents them from stimulating the impaired smell organ or its nerve branches. It may also help dysosmia that occurs out of the blue and without a trigger smell.

PRESCRIPTION MEDICATIONS. Gabapentin (Neurontin) and zonisamide (Zone-gran) have been helpful in reducing or eliminating dysosmia. These drugs, approved for use in seizure disorders, are not U.S. Food and Drug Administration (FDA) approved for treatment of smell disorders. However, physicians are permitted to use drugs that are approved by the FDA for "off label" purposes—purposes for which doctors have observed the drug to work but that have not been validated in large research studies. These drugs seem to work by reducing abnormal electrical discharges coming from the injured smell organ. The usual dosage is up to 600 mg twice a day of gabapentin or 100 mg twice a day of zonisamide.

SURGICAL REMOVAL OF THE SMELL ORGAN IN THE NOSE. This is the last resort option and will result in partial loss of smell. It is an option to consider only when dysosmia does not respond to these other treatments and quality of life is seriously affected by frequent abnormal smells. An ENT specialist performs this surgery.

Annette, who experienced dysosmia after a weeklong viral infection and became fearful of going near coffee or cologne because of the way it now smelled to her, tried the first two of these treatments. After using 5 to 10 cc of regular saline in each nostril every four or five hours each day, she found that her dysosmia improved markedly within a week and a half. She continued to have some episodes of abnormal smell that continued to upset her, however, so in addition to the nasal drops, she was prescribed gabapentin (Neurontin), 300 mg, twice a day. After two weeks, she found that the foul smell had almost disappeared. She is now able to enjoy her morning coffee and her husband's cologne, although neither smell is as intense as before. Even though food still does not taste normal, she is elated that her dysosmia is nearly gone. She can eat again without fear of bad smells. She is still taking gabapentin, because when she tries to decrease or eliminate it, the dysosmia returns. Her physician believes that she will eventually recover and no longer need the medication.

Dysosmia is not only very unpleasant; it can also (rarely) be life-threatening.

Seventy-five-year-old David began smelling a very foul odor whenever he came in contact with any foods he tried to eat. The smell was so bad, he almost stopped eating entirely. He lost 70 pounds in 3 months, became very weak and almost bedridden, and required stomach and intravenous feeding tubes to keep him alive. He was treated with a combination of intranasal saline solution, as previously described, and gabapentin tablets that were put in his stomach along with tube feedings. One week later, he noted the foul smells had decreased, and he began to eat vegetables, soups, and other liquids by mouth. He has continued to put on weight and is able to swallow an increasing variety of foods. The cause of his smell loss and severe dysosmia remains unknown, but happily he is improving. If he did not respond to this treatment program, serious consideration would have been given to removing his smell organ entirely.

Abnormal Levels of Vitamins and Hormones

If the cause of a taste and smell problem is unclear, most physicians will check the levels of thyroid hormone, vitamin B_{12}, and zinc through blood tests. Although there are no specific, unique smell and taste symptoms that particularly point to problems with thyroid hormone or levels of vitamin B_{12} and zinc, it is generally agreed that since these abnormalities are easily treated, they are worth testing in most cases of smell and taste impairment.

Low levels of vitamin B_{12} and zinc are usually due to impaired absorption in the stomach and small bowel, which can be caused by thinning of the stomach lining with aging, frequent use of medication to reduce stomach acid (heartburn), and diseases of the stomach and small bowel that cause prolonged nausea and vomiting, decreased appetite, and weight loss. Zinc deficiency, in addition to impairing the function of the taste receptor cells, plays a special role in taste disorders because it impairs the action of saliva from breaking down food we eat, which is necessary to stimulate the taste receptors so we can appreciate the basic tastes.

If low zinc or vitamin B_{12} levels or an underactive thyroid are considered the cause of smell and taste problems, these conditions can often be remedied. Vitamin B_{12} can be increased by injections of vitamin B_{12}; zinc levels can be increased by use of zinc tablets (zinc gluconate); and low thyroid levels can be normalized by thyroid supplement medication. Routine use of zinc tablets has not been shown to improve smell and taste abnormalities, however, unless the zinc level is low.

Simply eating foods rich in zinc and vitamin B_{12}—for example, high protein foods such as meats—or taking supplement tablets is unlikely to compensate for the low levels because these methods of delivery are not absorbed well by the body. Instead, injections of large amounts of vitamin B_{12} enter directly into the bloodstream and correct the low level in a short time. High doses of specific zinc gluconate tablets can also raise a low zinc level that cannot otherwise be raised.

After treatment, smell and taste loss due to these disorders can take more than three months to improve because of the gradual way the nerve cell machinery of the smell and taste system recovers.

Smoking

Over a period of years, smoking can cause very mild smell and taste impairment. It has been shown to lower the UPSIT score by four points. Smokers with smell and taste disorders usually have additional factors that add to their smell loss from smoking, such as medications, aging, and, poor oral hygiene. Smell and taste alteration from smoking begins to recover when smoking is discontinued but could take as many years to return to normal as the number of years spent smoking.

Diabetes

As explained in Chapter 1, people with diabetes sometimes experience problems with their senses of smell and taste. Usually, smell and taste symptoms will diminish or resolve when diabetes is under control, so consider smell and taste problems potential warning signs that you should pay careful attention to diabetes management, and consult your physician.

> This was the case with Genevieve, the woman who experienced a strange, sweet, metallic taste in her mouth that never went away except when she was chewing food. It turned out that prior to developing this symptom, called dysgeusia, she had been having numbness, tingling, and burning in her feet and hands for over a year—classic signs of diabetic peripheral neuropathy (nerve damage leading to numbness, tingling, or pain, often in the hands and feet).
>
> Her doctor, who was not aware of the connection between smell and taste problems and diabetes, managed the neuropathy with small doses of a medication called gabapentin (Neurontin), but Genevieve also wanted relief from the strange taste. Doctors at a smell and taste clinic recommended sugar-free gum and sugar-free hard candy, which would allow her to occupy her mouth and tongue and stimulate the taste system in a manner similar to eating—but without eating an unhealthy amount of food. The gum and candy eliminated the bad taste. One month later, Genevieve noticed the dysgeusia was gradually improving, and by the end of the second month it was gone. The gum and candy provided symptomatic relief but had nothing to do with her recovery. Many diabetic nerve disorders are fleeting and can improve on their own.

Nasal Polyps and Other Growths

Nasal polyps, benign tumors, inflammatory disorders, and cancer of the nose can cause smell loss with or without nasal blockage. These growths can be seen on a CT scan of the nose and sinuses but are best evaluated—and, if necessary, biopsied or removed—by nasal endoscopy, a procedure done by ENT and throat specialists. When nasal polyps and benign tumors are surgically removed, smell loss can be improved or even returned to normal. Nasal cancers and inflammatory growths may require radiation therapy, chemotherapy, or antibiotics; treatment may improve smell loss.

Digestive Issues

Gastroesophageal reflux disease (GERD), also known as heartburn or acid indigestion that can cause a metallic or sour taste, can be improved by use of antacids, such as Maalox, Mylanta, or Pepto–Bismol, which buffer stomach acid. Pills that reduce acid production by the stomach, such as Nexium, Pepcid AC, and Zantac, may also be used.

Bell's Palsy

Taste loss due to Bell's palsy is usually very mild because it occurs on only one side of the tongue, on the same side as the facial paralysis. Remember that there are numerous taste receptors in the palate, on the normal unaffected side of the tongue and in the back of the throat that tend to make up for the taste receptors impaired in Bell's palsy. The taste loss usually resolves on its own in two to three months.

Seizures

Remember from Chapter 1 and Chapter 2 that smell and taste auras due to seizure activity in the brain are caused by short electrical discharges from the smell or taste region, lasting usually less than a few minutes. The smell or taste sensation is usually very unpleasant (for example, a burning rubber smell or metallic taste), followed by loss of consciousness and shaking and jerking of the whole body or just shaking and jerking on one side of the body without loss of consciousness.

Smell and taste auras due to seizures usually improve or disappear when antiseizure medications such as phenytoin (Dilantin) or carbamazepine (Tegretol) are given.

Insufficient Saliva

Insufficient saliva (dry mouth) due to any one of a number of conditions can affect the taste of food. Among the most common causes are prescription medications that block saliva release. Saliva released from the salivary glands depends on a neurotransmitter called acetylcholine. Some medications block acetylcholine release and saliva diminishes.

The medications most commonly linked to this phenomenon are amitriptyline (Elavil), paroxetine (Paxil), and tolterodine (Detrol). The first two are antidepressants; the last one is used to reduce bladder urgency and frequent urination.

A number of treatment options are available for inadequate saliva. Artificial saliva is available from most drugstores without a prescription; these preparations have no side effects. Look for names such as Xero-Lube, Mouth Kote, and Saliva Substitute. They are placed in the mouth and tongue just before mealtime to help dissolve the food particles.

If artificial saliva does not help your dry mouth and improve the taste of your food, your doctor can prescribe a medication called pilocarpine in tablet form to be taken a few times a day. It stimulates acetylcholine release in the body and salivary gland. Unlike artificial saliva, however, this medication does occasionally come with side effects, such as muscle and abdominal cramps, sweating, and frequent urination. These side effects can sometimes be reduced by taking lower doses of the medication.

Living Well with a Smell and Taste Disorder

Staying Safe

Smell and taste disorders aren't just irritations or inconveniences that get in the way of our enjoyment of food. They can put your health and safety at risk. If you have been diagnosed with a smell and taste disorder, you should be aware of many potential hazards. To prevent injury and promote health and hygiene, remember these key tips:

Tips for Staying Safe and Healthy with a Smell or Taste Disorder

1. Be sure to have working smoke detectors and a natural gas or propane monitor in your home. Change the batteries on these monitors regularly (for instance, whenever you turn the clocks forward or back for daylight saving time).

2. Date all perishable foods and refrigerate them to prevent accidental food poisoning. Many foods can be spoiled before there are visible signs.

3. Label and store all garden products and household cleaning products properly. You don't want to mix up bug killer with fertilizer—or even more dangerously—window cleaner with fruit punch.

4. Be extra attentive while cooking to prevent burned food or a possible fire. Someone with a keen sense of smell may be able to leave a pot on the stove or a pan of brownies in the oven; they will be alerted by the aroma if something starts to burn. If you have a smell impairment, it's better to stay in the kitchen.

5. Bathe and shower regularly, and wash or dry clean clothes on a regular basis. Use underarm deodorant regularly. Use perfume and other fragrances sparingly, and check with family or friends to be sure you are not overdoing it.

6. If you care for young children, be sure to monitor frequently for diaper changes. The traditional mom's "sniff test" won't work for you!

Fixing Your Food

For most people, the most troublesome part of having a smell and taste disorder is related to the enjoyment of food and drink. It is frustrating to be unable to savor the sweetness and flavor of ice cream or the rich aroma of coffee in the morning. Even if you never completely recover from your smell and taste disorder, you can have much of that enjoyment back with a new awareness about food preparation.

Food preparation is one of the most important remedies for smell and taste disorders, regardless of the cause. It can help improve appetite and nutrition, maintain weight, and make eating more enjoyable. Even if you have a treatable smell and taste loss, changes in food preparations are important until you recover.

If your sense of smell and taste is severely impaired, you might wonder how much can be done to help you enjoy your food again. Consider the results of just one study, published in 2007.[2] This study evaluated the effects of nutritional education and flavor enhancement for cancer patients with impaired smell and taste. (Cancer patients may experience loss of smell and taste following chemotherapy and radiation therapy.) Half received nutritional information only, while the other half also received flavor enhancement products and foods such as bacon bits, sun-dried tomatoes, bananas, pear nectar, butter, and cheese extracts, which could be added to their foods to improve flavor. They were also shown how the flavors and foods could be used and combined.

This group was also educated in how to chew their food well to increase salivation and allow aromas and food molecules to travel up the back of the nose to the smell organ. They were encouraged to move their tongues around to push the foods to the soft palate, which has many taste buds. They also were told to prepare and eat foods that are crispy, crunchy, and chewy, and to vary the temperature to stimulate the trigeminal system.

At the end of eight months, the group receiving education and flavor enhancement had greater improvement in smell and taste perception and a slightly better quality of life. Their smell and taste had not actually changed—tests showed no difference—but their perception of improved smell and taste was notable.

Patients who received educational information about nutrition and flavor enhancement, recipes, and food preparation tips from a smell and taste clinic also reported having a better quality of life.

So are you ready to improve your next meal? Here are some key principles behind adding spice to your food and back into your life!

Top Tips for Enhancing Taste

1. Choose foods with varying colors and textures. For example, plain consommé soups can be replaced with tortilla soup, which has increased thickness, crunchy texture, and various spices, as well as different-colored vegetables to give more taste appeal. It emphasizes texture, temperature, and spicy and salty tastes. Bake fish filets a bit longer so the outside is crunchier. Grill hot dogs longer so they are crunchier, and serve them with blue corn chips, which have more appeal to some than plain corn chips.

2. Add spicy condiments, like peppers, horseradish, mustard, or salsa.

3. Increase the flavor of fish, poultry, and meat by marinating in sweet fruit juices, sweet wine, sweet and sour sauce, or spicy salad dressing.

4. Increase the savory taste of meats and poultry by using small amounts of MSG.

5. Serve foods hot and steaming to allow the aroma to fill the dining area.

6. Chew slowly, and move food slowly around your mouth in order to stimulate all your taste and sensory receptors.

7. Alternate bites of different foods during the meal.

8. Eat tart foods such as oranges and grapefruits, and drink tart beverages such as lemonade and grapefruit juice with their pulp. Remember, the ability to taste sweet and sour is usually normal in the majority of people with taste and smell loss.

Personalized Food Enhancement Plans

If you have a smell and taste disorder you are likely to fit into one of the three following categories. These categories are based on symptoms and test results. For each of these three categories, particular strategies can be employed to maximize your enjoyment of food and drink.

Partial Smell Loss with Normal Basic Taste (Sweet, Sour, Bitter, Salty, and Umami) and Normal Trigeminal Function (Texture, Temperature, and Spice)

Individuals in this category are able to detect most flavors and can perceive the temperature, texture, and spiciness of food, but because of partial smell loss they are likely to need higher concentrations of flavors. The most common reason for this kind of disorder is simply normal aging. Others causes include chronic sinus infections, allergies with nasal congestion, viral infections, and medications. Neurologic disorders such as Alzheimer's disease, Parkinson's disease, and multiple sclerosis may also result in partial smell loss.

A natural inclination may be to douse foods with salt or sugar to compensate for the loss of flavor. That may work, but it can also lead to hypertension or diabetes. Artificial sweeteners, salt substitutes, or MSG (for example, lower-sodium Accent) should be tried instead of regular sugar and salt. There are many artificial and natural flavors you can add to food to improve flavor. These are described in Chapter 6. When you use these flavor additives, start with twice the normal concentration and adjust up or down according to your preferences.

Some of you may be wondering about the safety of using artificial flavors, sugar substitutes, and MSG instead of regular salt. To date, no documented scientific evidence exists that proves these substitutes are harmful to humans. Most people with diabetes are familiar with artificial sweeteners and use them in cooking and baking; they are available in many processed foods in the diabetic section in grocery stores. There are also plenty of natural flavor products one can purchase at the grocery store.

MSG has had a long history of reported side effects, which has made many people unnecessarily fearful of using it in their food. Although MSG has clearly been shown to trigger migraine headaches in some people prone to them already, and can cause congestion, a runny nose, and allergy-like symptoms in others, such side effects are much less common than many people think. Remember that a lot of natural products that we eat contain high levels of MSG. Tomatoes, cheddar cheese, and scallops are a few that you likely have not had a problem eating.

If MSG has caused or worsened your migraines or has produced an allergic-type reaction, such as stuffy nose, congestion, and tearing of the eyes, you should avoid using it in food preparation; otherwise, there is little reason to fear MSG. Keep in mind that regular MSG has the same sodium content as table salt; if you have high blood pressure, a kidney disorder, or any other reason for maintaining low salt levels, try using a low-sodium MSG substitute called Accent. Substitute salt is potassium chloride, which is not a basic tastant like umami (savory) and will not help your food taste better. In fact, it has a bitter, metallic taste.

Moderate to Severe Smell Loss with Normal Basic Taste and Trigeminal Function

Individuals in this category are unlikely to be able to detect flavors, although the basic tastes (sweet, sour, salty, bitter, and umami) and trigeminal functions, such as the ability to detect temperature, texture, and spice, are normal. Most often this type of smell impairment is due to brain and nasal trauma, viral infections, certain medications, or exposure to certain chemicals and toxins. Marked smell loss can also be seen in certain neurologic disorders such as Alzheimer's disease and Parkinson's disease. Emphasizing food appearance, texture, and temperature and using spices and basic tastes is helpful.

Adding natural or artificial flavors may not always be helpful, but they are worthwhile to try since although most people with moderate smell loss lose the ability to detect most flavors (such as strawberry or vanilla), this does not happen to everyone.

Normal Smell and Trigeminal Function with Altered Basic Taste

Depending on the severity of the taste loss, individuals in this category usually have some difficulty recognizing flavors because of altered taste, but flavor loss is usually less severe than in primary smell disorders. This type of impairment is less common than the other categories and is rarely severe. Common causes include heavy smoking; poor oral and dental hygiene; ill-fitting dentures; saliva deficiency; some medications; and dietary deficiencies of vitamin B_6, vitamin B_{12}, calcium, or zinc. Severe taste loss may occur with radiation therapy for cancer of the head and neck. Also, normal aging results in mild basic taste impairment, especially for sweet and salt.

Changes in food preparation should include adding spices and higher concentrations of flavors and tastants. Again, salt and sugar should be used with care because of the risk of high blood pressure and diabetes. Artificial sweeteners and small amounts of MSG (for example, lower-sodium Accent) can substitute for sugar and table salt.

Counseling

The enjoyment of food and pleasant aromas are an important part of the human experience. How often do we tell family and friends about the wonderful meal we had at a fine restaurant? These are ordinary pleasures of life that we often take for granted—until they are impaired or gone. In a 2001 study of people with smell and taste disorders, more than half of the participants said they would be willing to spend more than one-fifth of their annual income to successfully treat their conditions.[3] Not surprisingly, when we suddenly find such simple but essential experiences taken away from us, it's not unusual to become depressed.

Depression occurs in about one-third to one-half of people with smell and taste disorders. It is usually mild but can be severe. Many people who experience depression improve when they understand more about their particular problem and learn ways to cope with it. Others may benefit from psychological counseling and antidepressant medications. As with many chronic disorders, forming support groups and exchanging recipes—such as those found in this book—with others who have similar problems can be reassuring and helpful.

Potential New Treatments

Promising new treatments are currently being developed for smell and taste disorders. Researchers at the University of Dresden Medical School in Germany are studying "odor training" to help people with smell impairment.[4] Patients are given samples of pleasant odors that they smell twice a day for 12 weeks. Each odor is sniffed for two seconds and repeated twice in each session. Each session lasts two minutes. Results seem to suggest overall improvement in smell function, especially for the odors used in the trials. Further research is needed to learn more about this promising new approach.

Another study from 2005 is based on the interesting role that calcium plays in our normal smell function.[5] Mucus secreted during the normal smell process has a high calcium concentration that helps to reduce the duration of the electrical discharge of the olfactory nerve cell so the odor that is recognized is not noticed after a short while.

(This is part of the reason why you may not notice the smell of a strong perfume or a dirty diaper as much after you've been in the room with the scent for awhile.) These studies show that changing the calcium content of nasal mucus may help improve smell function.

One of these studies evaluated smell function before and after introducing a sodium citrate buffer solution in the nose. The purpose of the buffer solution was to lower the calcium content of the mucus so that the olfactory nerve cells would continue to discharge and recognize the odors. Almost everyone who participated had improved smell scores on testing in less than one hour. Subjectively, three-fourths of the participants reported their smell improved for up to three hours after the use of the buffer solution. Although this approach sounds promising, the study was preliminary, and therapies aimed at calcium content in the nasal mucus will need to be evaluated further.

Looking to the Future

Our understanding of the structure and function of the smell and taste system has come a long way, especially since the last quarter of the twentieth century. The development of standardized smell testing and improved taste testing, along with improved imaging (MRI and CT scans) and advances in biochemistry and genetics, have all allowed us to better understand the natural history of smell and taste changes in the normal aging population and in disorders of smell and taste.

These advances have also been instrumental in helping physicians identify disorders of smell and taste in patients with Parkinson's disease, multiple sclerosis, and certain dementias such as Alzheimer's disease and dementia with Lewy bodies that may not be recognized by the patients and their caregivers. These patients, in the course of their illnesses, often develop decreased appetite, weight loss, and depression due to problems with smell and taste, which are often falsely thought to be caused by more serious medical conditions, such as cancer and gastrointestinal disorders. The future shows great promise in many aspects of smell and taste. Currently some evidence suggests that smell testing in the normal population has been of some help in predicting who may possibly develop amnestic mild cognitive impairment and who is likely to develop Alzheimer's disease. Research in the future may well incorporate smell testing alongside other tests, such as measuring brain volume with MRI scan and analyzing spinal fluid, to make a more accurate and early diagnosis of dementia, especially Alzheimer's disease. Smell testing has already been accepted by the American Academy of Neurology as helpful in distinguishing typical Parkinson's disease from the atypical varieties. Since smell testing is neither invasive nor expensive and is very easy to administer, it offers an excellent alternative to help diagnose many of these troubling neurologic conditions.

For the past 50 years, it has been known that smell and taste receptor cells regularly divide and renew themselves. More research is needed to see if this capability can be used to improve smell and taste disorders and make renewed effective connections to the smell and taste system.

More work is needed to identify more recipes and further changes in food preparation to positively impact the lives of people with these disorders. This change in food preparation information needs to be taught to health care providers and expanded to nutritionists, dieticians, and the culinary and restaurant professions.

Rapidly expanding information on the genetics of olfactory receptors initially identified by 2004 Nobel prize winners Drs. Linda B. Buck and Richard Axel will continue to give us insight into how the smell system works, and hopefully will lead to better treatments.

References

1. Geha RS, Beiser A, Ren C, et al. Review of alleged reaction to monosodium glutamate and outcome of a multicenter double-blind placebo-controlled study. *Journal of Nutrition* 2000;130:1058S–1062S.

This article dispels some myths about MSG. It is generally very safe and only on occasion can give some mild reactions.

2. Schiffman SS, Sattely-Miller EA, Taylor EL, et al. Combination of flavor enhancement and chemosensory education improves nutritional status in older cancer patients. *Journal of Nutrition, Health and Aging* 2007;11(5): 439–454.

This detailed article on flavor enhancement and education about the smell and taste impairment in cancer patients supports the idea that education and changes in food preparation are very helpful in improving quality of life.

3. Miwa T, Furukawa M, Tsukatani T, et al. Impact of olfactory impairment on quality of life and disability. *Archives of Otolaryngology–Head and Neck Surgery* 2001;127:497–503.

This article describes in detail how quality of life in a large study population can be seriously impaired by smell and taste loss.

4. Hummel T, Rissom K, Reden J, et al. Effects of olfactory training in patients with olfactory loss. *Laryngoscope* 2009;119(3): 496–499.

This article describes the treatment of repeatedly smelling different odors to try to improve olfactory function. This study suggested some possible improvement, but more work is needed to confirm this treatment.

5. Panagiotopoulos G, Naxakis S, Papavasiliou A. Decreasing nasal mucous Ca++ improves hyposmia. *Rhinology* 2005;43(2):130–134.

This study changed the calcium content of the mucus of the upper nose by using a buffer solution, which created short-term improvement in smell. This is a very promising therapy, but more work is needed to prolong the effects of the buffer solution; many more people with smell and taste impairment must be tested to determine who improves and for how long.

6

Food Preparation

In this chapter, you'll learn:

▶ Detailed tips for food preparation

▶ Flavoring options

▶ How to prepare flavorful recipes customized for people with smell and taste disorders

General Information

Many patients with smell and taste disorders and their families have difficulty applying the important tips about food preparation to their daily routines. Some request step-by-step instructions, and others are confronted by the problem of preparing two different meals: one for the family member with smell and taste impairment and another for everybody else.

The solution? Recipes that are easily modified to suit everyone at the table. The recipes that follow this chapter were selected with the help of food adviser Marjorie Calvert and a professional chef. Combining their culinary expertise and experience with the special needs of people with smell and taste disorders, they discovered and developed recipes that emphasize texture, temperature, tartness, and spiciness—recipes that can be easily modified so that they enhance the dining experience of people with smell and taste disorders while not overwhelming the palates of everyone else at the table.

These recipes were tested by people spanning a wide age range and included those both with and without a smell and taste disorder. Most of those with smell and taste impairments had moderate to severe smell loss with the inability to detect flavors, but they had normal taste function (for sweet, sour, bitter, salty, and umami/savory) and normal trigeminal function (recognition of temperature, texture, and spice).

Recipes were prepared four different ways: first using the original unaltered recipe, and then three other ways with different concentrations of seasonings, such as ginger, vinegar, garlic, citrus, jalapeno peppers, cayenne pepper, and monosodium glutamate (MSG), depending on the particular recipe. The participants rated each portion based on two questions: (1) Did they enjoy the taste of this food? (2) Would they try this food preparation again?

Recipes that we tested are only included in this book if they received a minimum of a 50 percent approval rating by those with impaired smell and taste. The majority of the recipes received 75 to 100 percent approval. Most of the people with normal smell and taste function only enjoyed the original recipes, so the recipes included here are designed to be easily modifiable so that two entirely separate meals need not be prepared to make everyone at the table happy.

> In our practice we request that our patients fill out a questionnaire before their clinic visit that asks about their food likes and dislikes prior to and after their smell and taste problem began, including questions about preferences among spices, flavors, textures, and various foods such as fish, poultry, and meat. With this food preference information and the results of smell and taste testing, each person receives food recommendations that may be able to enhance his or her enjoyment of food and overall quality of life.

In addition to specific recipes, there are simple "tweaks" you can make to your usual dishes to help you enjoy your meals more. For example, if you have enjoyed eating lightly salted scrambled eggs with buttered toast and black coffee for breakfast, you will likely not enjoy it as much if you have smell and taste loss. The eggs and toast will have little to no flavor, but they will retain their texture and temperature. The coffee will retain temperature but will likely have no taste.

If your smell loss is mild and your taste and trigeminal function is normal, you might want to try different varieties of seasoned salt. Choose the salts you like and use them on your eggs. Adding chunky salsa to eggs instead can give you a spicy taste along with the texture of the vegetables in the salsa. You can enhance the butter flavor on your toast by using artificially flavored additives such as McCormick Butter Flavored Salt, Watkins Imitation Butter Flavored Salt, or any butter-flavored products you can find at the grocery store. You can also try adding fruit preserves to your toast for sweetness and texture. Enhancing the taste of black coffee is more of a challenge. You can try to make stronger coffee or perhaps consider adding a sweetener or flavored creamer for texture. Or instead of coffee, you might want to try a glass of cold orange or grapefruit juice with pulp for a sweet-tart taste and texture. If your smell loss is more severe, you might try many of the same changes, but some—such as the butter-flavored additives—might not be as helpful because more severe smell loss is likely to impair the ability to identify flavors of any kind.

Using Umami Compounds in Food Preparation

As previously mentioned, umami is one of the five basic tastes, which also include sweet, sour, bitter, and salt. Umami, a Japanese word, is roughly translated as "tasty" but has also more descriptively been translated as savory, meaty, or brothy. It enhances the savory flavor of food, increases palatability, and contributes to the sense of satisfaction and fullness after eating. Studies have also shown that umami increases salivary flow, which ensures that food particles are broken down in the mouth to release aromas. So for people with impaired smell or taste function, it makes sense to look at how to increase the presence of umami in foods that do not have it naturally. Fortunately, this taste can be added to many foods using the food additive MSG.

Umami occurs naturally in many foods, including meat, fish sauces, dairy products, and tomatoes. Bouillon cubes, shiitake mushrooms, and seaweed all have the main components of the ideal umami taste as well. In fact, the Swiss invented bouillon cubes in 1882 for people who could not afford meat but wanted to enjoy the same flavor and taste sensation.

This may not work for everyone, however. Up to one-fifth of the general population may not be able to taste umami due to genetic factors. And a very small percentage of the population may have side effects from MSG, including nasal congestion and mild headaches.

How much MSG is necessary in food preparation to achieve the umami taste? The suggested amount is 300 to 800 milligrams of MSG for each 100 grams of food, or ¼ to ½ teaspoon per 8 ounces of food. By using MSG (or Accent, which is a low-sodium form of MSG), you can reduce the amount of table salt needed in order to improve the enjoyment of food for someone with a smell and taste disorder. It's important to know that MSG normally has similar sodium content to table salt, especially if you or someone you are cooking for is elderly, has high blood pressure, or otherwise needs to limit salt intake.

There are also many foods that have a higher natural umami content, including tomatoes, corn, mushrooms, and cabbage. These vegetables, and other examples below, can be eaten in greater quantities to increase the umami taste, resulting in greater enjoyment of food. Other foods that contain high concentrations of naturally occurring umami are walnuts, Roquefort cheese, edamame, soy sauce, tofu, broccoli, sauerkraut, and dried beans. Below is a table of umami-rich foods and their natural umami concentrations by weight.

Natural Umami Concentration by Weight in Different Foods

Food	Milligrams per 100 Grams
Meat and Poultry	
Beef	10
Chicken	22
Seafood	
Scallop	140
Blue crab	43
Alaskan king crab	72
Shrimp (white)	20
Seaweed	
Kombu (dried seaweed)	1608
Vegetables	
Cabbage	50
Spinach	48
Tomato	246
Corn	106
Green peas	106
Potato	10
Shitake mushrooms (fresh)	71

Natural Umami Concentration by Weight in Different Foods (*continued*)

Food	Milligrams per 100 Grams
Fruits	
Avocado	18
Apple	4
Cheese	
Parmigiano Reggiano	1680
Cheddar	182
Milk	
Cow	1
Goat	4
Concentrated extracts	
Oyster sauce	900

In Chapter 5, we discussed the potential benefits of adding natural and/or artificial flavors to your food as a strategy to enhance palatability. Flavor enhancement may be helpful regardless of how severe the taste loss. You may want to start by sprinkling enough of the artificial flavor or extract to lightly cover the food. Increase or decrease the amount according to preference. All of the extracts and flavors listed below are available from many different manufacturers and can be found either at your local grocery or online.

Flavors and Extracts

Extracts and flavorings are used to give foods enhanced "taste interest" and more concentrated flavor. Try these extracts and flavorings in foods, sweets, and beverages.

Almond,
    Imitation
Almond, Pure
Amaretto
Anise, Pure
Apple
Apricot
Banana
Blackberry
Black Raspberry

Black Walnut
Blueberry
Bourbon
Brandy
Butter
Butter Pecan
Butterscotch
Caramel
Champagne
Cherry

Wild Cherry
Chocolate
Cinnamon
Coconut,
    Imitation
Coffee
Coffee Liqueur
Cotton Candy
Cream Soda
Elderberry

Egg Nog
Garlic
Grape
Hazelnut
Honey
Irish Cream
Key Lime
Lemon
Lime Twist
Macadamia Nut
Maple
Orange
Orange Liqueur
Passion Fruit

Peach
Pear
Pecan
Peanut Butter
Peppermint
Pina Colada
Pistachio
Pineapple
Plum
Pomegranate
Pumpkin Spice
Raspberry
Raspberry, Black
Root Beer

Rose Water
Rum
Sherry
Spearmint
Strawberry
Wild Strawberry
Vanilla Beans
Vanilla Butter & Nut
Vanilla Extract, Pure
Vanilla Extract,
   Imitation
Vanilla Extract, White
   (Clear)
Violet

Spice Up Your Popcorn

Try these seasonings on your next batch of popcorn. Popcorn should be hot and popped in oil for seasonings to stick.

▶ Barbecue
▶ Cheddar cheese
▶ Cheese and spice
▶ Chocolate caramel
▶ Dill pickle
▶ Kettle corn
▶ Nacho cheese

▶ Parmesan garlic
▶ Popcorn salt
▶ Ranch
▶ Salt and vinegar
▶ Sour cream and onion
▶ Southwest jalapeno
▶ White cheddar

Five Basic Tastes, Unlimited Flavors

See the list below for a few examples of the many different flavors that are derived from the five basic tastes. Use them in cooking and food preparation to enhance the aroma and taste of your food.

Sweet

Fruit juices and purees, bananas, strawberries, dates, figs, grapes, beets, carrots, corn, poppy seeds, sesame seeds, sesame oil, coriander, cilantro, honey, vanilla extract, peppermint extract, any nut extract, sweetened chocolate, milk chocolate, sugars and syrups of all sorts, molasses, sugar substitutes, sugar. *Many of these are available in sugar-free form for diabetics.*

Sour
All vinegars, vinegar-based dressings, lemons, limes, oranges, pineapple, apples, yogurt, yeast breads (sourdough), creamy salad dressings (Thousand Island, Ranch, Green Goddess), pickles, pickled foods, citric acid food additive.

Bitter
Coffee, beer, citrus peel, unsweetened chocolate, quinine (tonic water), Angostura bitters, cabbage, cauliflower, broccoli, turnips, spinach, radicchio, turnip greens, mustard greens, dandelion greens, lettuces, jicama, barley, horseradish, garlic, basil.

Salty
Table salt, cottage cheese, hard cheeses, most dairy products, frozen prepared foods, canned foods, pickles, chips and packaged snack foods, salted nuts, processed meat and fish (deli lunch meat, smoked salmon, pickled herring, canned tuna, sardines), shell fish, bottled salad dressings, ketchup, canned or bottled tomato sauce, soy sauce. *Those with high blood pressure should use the above items sparingly. Look for reduced sodium versions of these products.*

Umami (Savory)
Monosodium glutamate (MSG), liquid smoke, soy sauce, fish sauce, walnuts, grapes, broccoli, tomatoes, asparagus, corn, potatoes, soy beans (edamame), shiitake and other mushrooms, dried beans, meats, parmesan cheese, Roquefort cheese, fermented cabbage foods (sauerkraut, kimchi).

The table on the next page showing samples of food and spice combinations that can improve taste by increasing texture, temperature, spiciness, umami, and other basic tastes that are still recognized and appreciated in smell and taste loss. You may want to try many different spices with each food to find the combinations most pleasing to your palate.

Be creative and find what works for you!

Examples of Food and Spice Combinations That Can Improve Taste

Foods	Spice Combinations
Breads	Poppy seed, sesame seed, fennel seed, anise, caraway seed, dill, thyme, garlic, parsley
Vegetables	Tarragon, rosemary, parsley, oregano, marjoram, sage, garlic, thyme, dill, anise, basil
Beef	Tarragon, rosemary, dill, thyme, bay leaf, basil, oregano, marjoram, garlic
Poultry	Tarragon, parsley, sage, thyme, rosemary, caraway, oregano, basil, paprika, bay leaf
Pork	Rosemary, cumin, caraway seed, parsley. mustard, fennel seed, thyme, basil
Lamb	Thyme, dill, fennel seed, basil, sage, marjoram, tarragon, rosemary. caraway seed
Soups	Rosemary, dill, caraway seed, anise, parsley, sage, basil, bay leaf, oregano, chives, tarragon
Fish	Marjoram, tarragon, rosemary, bay leaf, basil, thyme, dill, sage
Shellfish	Oregano, basil, garlic salt, marjoram, thyme, dill, tarragon, turmeric
Eggs	Thyme, garlic, chives, bay leaf, oregano, dill, basil, parsley, rosemary, tarragon
Cheese	Anise, thyme, parsley, caraway seed, dill, sage, basil, tarragon
Desserts	Vanilla bean, anise, allspice, cinnamon, nutmeg

Food Preparation Methods Suggested by Patients with Smell and Taste Disorders

Following this chapter, we include many detailed recipes that were sent to us by many of our patients. We believe that if a person with smell and taste problems recommends a recipe or a modification to normal food preparation, this strongly suggests that many other people with the same problem will also find it helpful. Just a few of the many suggestions we have received from patients with smell and taste loss include:

▶ Char-grilled hamburgers (almost burned)
▶ Grilled salmon with chopped onions
▶ Grilled pork (almost burned)
▶ Barbecued chicken—save some BBQ sauce for extra dipping

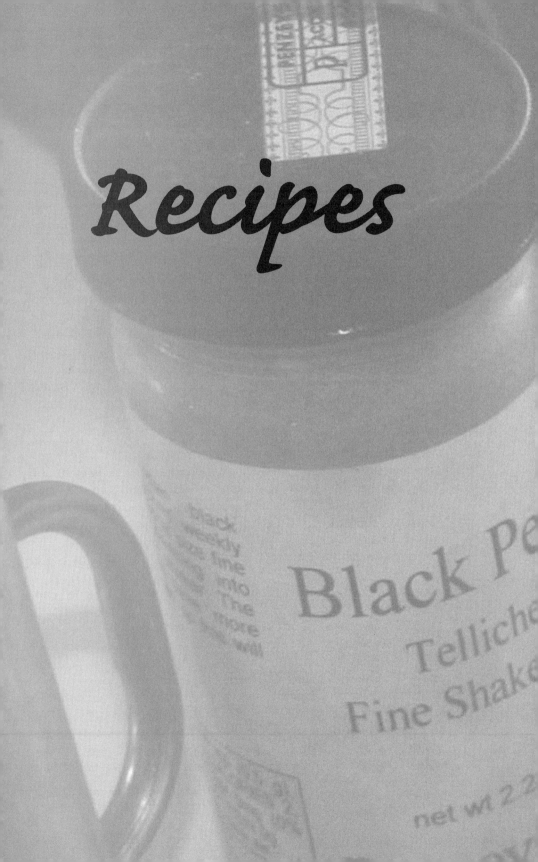

Recipes

Introduction

Whether you have smell and taste loss or normal smell and taste function, before you decide to prepare any of the following recipes, it is important to understand both why they are included and how successful they were in improving eating enjoyment.

From experience at our clinic and from reviewing many clinical research studies on smell and taste loss, we know that changes in food preparation are among the most important approaches to treatment. Most patients we see report that food tastes bad, has no taste at all, or that eating is no longer pleasurable or satisfying. If you have impaired smell or taste, it is helpful to be aware of tips for preparing foods you enjoyed prior to the smell and taste loss, such as adding more spice to foods with condiments like salsa, horseradish, or mustard and varying food texture and temperature. These tips are helpful because spicy foods stimulate the sensory nerve function of the trigeminal nerve, which usually continues to function normally in people with smell and taste disorders. Adding MSG (a umami, or savory, taste that is spared in most smell disorders) in a "pinch" quantity, or as much as an eighth of a teaspoon, through a low-sodium additive such as Accent to steak and chicken increases the savory taste of the meat. Chewing foods longer to stimulate the mouth's taste receptors fully can also be helpful in improving eating enjoyment.

We have found that many of our patients are not familiar with these basic food preparation tips. They also generally prefer not to have to make two different meals—for those with and those without smell and taste problems.

In 2004, along with sous chef Chris Lee, we discussed the feasibility of developing recipes to emphasize texture, temperature, spice, and taste (sweet, salty, umami, and sour). Marji and Chris came up with 18 recipes from a combination of personal experience and various cookbooks. As a pilot project, we tested these recipes with seven patients with a smell and/or taste disorder related to various causes, as well as three people with normal smell and taste. The 18 recipes were tested over two separate testing days, one week apart. None of the 10 individuals tested knew the specific ingredients contained in what they were eating. For each round of testing, one recipe was used. Four numbered samples were given to each person tested. One sample consisted of the original recipe and the other three samples consisted of the original recipe with one variation: an additional spice or tastant, such as jalapeño pepper, Tabasco sauce, ginger, or an MSG product such as Accent. At the end of each round, tasters were asked whether they enjoyed one or all variations of the single recipe and whether they would eat that sample again in the future. If 50 percent or more rated it favorably and said they would eat it again, then we accepted that recipe with its variation and distributed it to those tested to use at home. The same methodology was applied to all 18 recipes. In the end, only half of the original recipes and their variations were rated favorably enough to continue to recommend them. The subjects with no smell or taste impairment generally enjoyed the original recipes without variations (that is, the addition of spices, MSG, or other tastants).

This chapter includes the recipes that emerged from our pilot testing, as well as other recipes that were submitted to us by individuals with smell and taste disorders. Recipes that have a *variation box* included with the main recipe are the ones we tested in our study that were found to be favorable additions by those with a smell and/or taste disorder. If you decide to use these recipes and want to try a variation, choose only one variation at a time. Some people with smell and taste impairment may actually find the original recipe enjoyable without any changes. This is something with which you will need to experiment. Since the variations in the boxes next to the recipes are often unlikely to be enjoyed by those with normal smell and taste, we recommend preparing the recipe without variation for the whole family and experimenting with adding one variation at a time to enhance the portion served to those with problems with smell and taste.

The recipes that do not have variation boxes were submitted by our patients. We did not specifically test these recipes with other patients. Since individuals with smell and taste impairment enjoyed these recipes enough to bring them to us, we believe others will enjoy them as well.

Following each recipe, we describe the preparation time and the level of difficulty to prepare (easy, moderately challenging, or challenging).

Positive feedback from our study participants led us to add education on food preparation to our patients' routine visits to our clinic. We also began to distribute popular recipes to our patients and to offer taste samples of selected spices and salts to demonstrate that changes in food preparation may result in greater enjoyment of food and improved appetite.

In 2008 we conducted a follow-up telephone survey with 40 patients we had assessed in the clinic over the previous three years. We also surveyed 45 patients we had seen prior to 2005, before we were providing education about food preparation and distributing recipes. Seventy percent of the group of patients seen after 2005 was satisfied with the information they received about food preparation. The majority of this group was still using the recipes and food preparation tips at the time of the survey, whether they had recovered from their smell and taste disorder or not. On the other hand, only 30 percent of the group of patients seen by us prior to 2005 was satisfied with the information they received about food preparation. This survey taught us how important food preparation information is in the management of smell and taste disorders.

The recipes suggested in this section of the book may not satisfy everyone. We all have different opinions about food. We recommend that you experiment with these recipes and find the ones that work best for you and your family. Our experience shows that when individuals with a smell and taste disorder find a recipe they like, it is more than likely that the recipe will also be enjoyed by family members and friends with normal smell and taste.

salads

- ▸ Asian Chicken Salad
- ▸ Chicken Salad with Grapes and Walnuts
- ▸ Curried Chicken Salad
- ▸ Spicy Thai Beef Salad

Asian Chicken Salad

Serves 4 to 6 | Preparation time: 45 minutes | Easy

This salad was chosen because of its good texture and the presence of both spices (hot red pepper flakes and Dijon mustard) and umami taste (soy sauce) in the vinaigrette. Only the standard recipe was tested—and enjoyed—by those with normal smell and taste. The first two variations shown in the box were enjoyed by 75 percent of those with smell and taste loss while the last variation was enjoyed by everyone with smell and taste loss.

INGREDIENTS

Vinaigrette
½ cup soy sauce
3 tablespoons seasoned rice vinegar
3 tablespoons vegetable oil
2 tablespoons Asian sesame oil
2 tablespoons Dijon mustard
2 tablespoons peeled, finely grated, fresh ginger
2 teaspoons dried hot red pepper flakes

Salad
4 cups coarsely shredded cooked chicken
3½ cups (½ pound) Napa cabbage, cut into 1-inch pieces
¼ pound snow peas, cut diagonally into 1-inch pieces
1 seedless cucumber, quartered lengthwise and cut into ½-inch pieces
3 scallions, finely chopped
½ cup chopped fresh cilantro

PREPARATION

Whisk together all vinaigrette ingredients and set aside. Combine salad ingredients in a large bowl and toss with vinaigrette until combined well.

> ### Vinaigrette Variations to Enhance Smell and Taste
> TRY ADDING: 1½ tablespoons seasoned rice vinegar *or* 1 tablespoon tarragon *or* 1½ teaspoons salt

Chicken Salad with Grapes and Walnuts

Serves 4 to 6 | Preparation time: 20–30 minutes | Easy

This recipe was chosen because of the varied texture provided by the chicken, walnuts, and celery; and the use of spices (vinegar, chopped tarragon, and black pepper), and salt. One hundred percent of our smell and taste-impaired tasters enjoyed the first two boxed variations and 75 percent enjoyed the third variation.

INGREDIENTS

4 cups cooked chicken, cubed in ½-inch pieces
1 cup toasted, chopped walnuts
1 cup celery, cut into ¼-inch-thick slices
2 tablespoons finely chopped shallot
2 cups halved seedless red grapes
1 cup mayonnaise
4 tablespoons vinegar
3 tablespoons finely chopped tarragon
⅔ tablespoon salt
⅔ teaspoon black pepper

PREPARATION

Toss all ingredients in a large bowl until combined well.

Variations to Enhance Smell and Taste
TRY ADDING: 1½ table-spoons vinegar *or* 1 tablespoon tarragon *or* 1½ teaspoons salt

Curried Chicken Salad

Serves 5 to 8 | Preparation time: 2½ hours | Easy

This recipe, which features interesting texture, spice (Asian chili paste and Dijon mustard), and strong basic taste (juice of 5 limes), was very popular among our tasters. One hundred percent of tasters with smell or taste impairment enjoyed the standard recipe and all the variations. Those with normal smell and taste enjoyed the standard recipe as well as the first variation with additional yellow curry powder.

INGREDIENTS

2 to 3 pounds boneless, skinless chicken breast
3 tablespoons yellow curry powder
Juice of 5 limes
1 each of yellow, green, and red peppers, diced
½ cup chopped, toasted pecans
1 bunch cilantro, chopped
4 ounces unsweetened coconut milk
½ cup Dijon mustard
2 tablespoons Asian chili paste
1 to 2 cups mayonnaise (depending on desired consistency)
Salt to taste
Cracked pepper to taste

PREPARATION

Marinate chicken breasts in curry powder and lime juice for 1 hour. Grill chicken and allow to cool for 1 hour. Once cool, dice chicken into ½-inch cubes. Place chicken in a mixing bowl and add diced peppers, pecans, cilantro, coconut milk, mustard, chili paste, and mayonnaise. Mix well and season with salt and pepper to taste. Serve chilled.

Variations to Enhance Smell and Taste

TRY ADDING: 1 teaspoon yellow curry powder *or* 1 ounce unsweetened coconut milk *or* 1 teaspoon Asian chili paste

Spicy Thai Beef Salad

Serves 4 | Preparation time: 30 minutes | Easy

One hundred percent of our tasters with smell and taste impairment enjoyed this recipe with extra lime juice or extra MSG (such as Accent). Fifty percent enjoyed extra sugar.

INGREDIENTS
7 tablespoons fresh lime juice
6 tablespoons Asian fish sauce
3 Thai chilies, minced
2 teaspoons sugar
½ pound thinly sliced rare beef
5 small scallions, cut into 1-inch lengths
3 medium shallots, thinly sliced
1 cup thinly sliced, peeled cucumber
½ cup chopped celery leaves

PREPARATION
In a large bowl, mix the lime juice, fish sauce, chilies, and sugar until sugar is dissolved. Add the beef, scallions, shallots, cucumber, and celery leaves. Toss gently and serve.

> **Variations to Enhance Smell and Taste**
> TRY ADDING: 1 tablespoon lime juice *or* 1½ teaspoon sugar *or* ¼ teaspoon MSG (such as Accent)

Sides

- ▸ *Green Chili Ginger Rice*
- ▸ *Horseradish Potatoes*
- ▸ *Mushroom Medley with Ginger, Garlic, and Soy*
- ▸ *"Pickled" Cucumbers and Onions*
- ▸ *Sautéed Mushrooms*

Green Chili Ginger Rice

Serves 4 | Preparation time: 45 minutes | Easy

This recipe was chosen for its good texture (white rice and bell peppers) and spice (ginger, garlic, and chili). We found that even those without smell and taste impairment enjoyed the extra garlic in the second variation. Seventy-five percent of our tasters with smell and taste impairment enjoyed the standard recipe and both variations.

INGREDIENTS

1 tablespoon vegetable oil
1 small onion, diced
1 cup uncooked long-grain white rice
1 tablespoon minced garlic
¼ cup finely chopped red bell pepper
¼ cup canned or fresh, diced green chilies
¼ cup sour cream
1½ cups water
3 teaspoons peeled, finely chopped, fresh ginger
1 teaspoon salt

PREPARATION

Heat vegetable oil in a 2- or 3-quart heavy saucepan over medium-high heat until hot but not smoking. Sauté onion, stirring until golden, about 5 minutes. Stir in remaining ingredients and bring to a boil. Reduce heat to low and cook, covered, for 15 minutes. Remove from heat and fluff with a fork.

Variations to Enhance Smell and Taste
TRY ADDING: 1½ teaspoons green chilies *or* ½ teaspoon minced garlic

Horseradish Potatoes

Serves 4 | Preparation time: 30 minutes | Easy

This recipe came to us highly recommended by a patient with impaired smell. We have shared it with many of our patients and the feedback has been very positive. The mixture of spice (horseradish) with texture (potatoes) along with other ingredients such as lemon juice (tart taste) has been popular with many, especially those who enjoy the taste of horseradish.

INGREDIENTS

¼ cup butter or margarine
1 tablespoon prepared horseradish
2 teaspoons lemon juice
½ teaspoon salt
⅛ teaspoon pepper
12 small new potatoes, cut in half

PREPARATION

Place butter or margarine in a microwave-safe, 1-quart dish. Microwave uncovered on high for 40 seconds, or until butter or margarine is melted. Stir in horseradish, lemon juice, salt, pepper, and potatoes. Cover and microwave on high for 10 minutes, stirring once. Let stand for 2 minutes and stir a final time before serving.

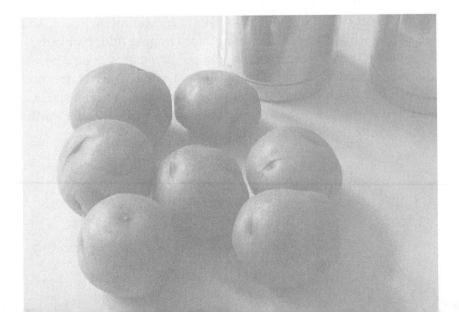

Mushroom Medley with Ginger, Garlic, and Soy

Serves 4 | Preparation time: 45 minutes | Moderately challenging

This recipe comes highly recommended by one of our patients. This colorful and delicious dish has a wonderful array of texture, spice, and basic tastes and is a perfect side for fish, meat, or poultry.

INGREDIENTS

2 teaspoons sesame oil
1 red bell pepper, cut into strips
2 tablespoons minced fresh ginger
1½ tablespoons minced garlic
8 ounces shiitake mushrooms, stems trimmed, caps sliced
8 ounces sliced button mushrooms
4 ounces small oyster mushrooms
1 10-ounce package spinach leaves, stems trimmed
6 green onions, cut into thin strips
1 tablespoon soy sauce
Salt
Pepper
4 lemon wedges

PREPARATION

Heat sesame oil in a large nonstick skillet over medium-high heat. Add bell pepper, ginger, and garlic and sauté for 1 minute. Add shiitake, button, and oyster mushrooms and sauté about 10 minutes, or until brown and tender, adding 2 to 3 tablespoons water if mixture is dry. Add spinach and green onions and stir about 2 minutes, or until spinach wilts. Stir in soy sauce. Season with salt and pepper. Transfer mushroom mixture to serving bowl and serve with lemon wedges.

"Pickled" Cucumbers and Onions

Serves 6 | Preparation time: 20 minutes | Easy

Another great recipe from one of our patients. The apple cider vinegar in combination with onions and cucumbers served cold gives a unique taste that is especially appreciated by people with smell and taste impairment.

INGREDIENTS
3 large cucumbers, thinly sliced
1 to 2 medium Vidalia or Texas 1015 onions, thinly sliced
Coarsely ground black pepper
Kosher or sea salt
1 32-ounce bottle apple cider vinegar
Ice cubes

PREPARATION
Slice cucumbers and onions as thin as possible and layer in a large, nonaluminum bowl with a cover. Add salt and pepper to taste between each layer. Fill bowl with apple cider vinegar until cucumber and onion slices are covered. Add ice cubes to cover surface area of bowl, leaving room to cover. Leave mixture at room temperature until ice cubes have melted. Stir well and place in refrigerator for several hours before serving.

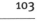

Sautéed Mushrooms

Serves 2 | Preparation time: 20 minutes | Easy

A recipe submitted by one of our patients, these mushrooms make a wonderful side dish for just about anything. If the standard recipe is not appreciated, try increasing the amount of soy sauce (umami) and/or lemon juice (sour, tart) to enhance its enjoyment for those with smell and taste impairment.

INGREDIENTS
2 tablespoons olive oil
10 ounces quartered mushrooms
1 tablespoon unsalted butter
2 cloves garlic, chopped
1 tablespoon fresh lemon juice
½ tablespoon soy sauce
1 teaspoon sugar

PREPARATION
Heat a 12-inch heavy skillet over moderately high heat until very hot. Add olive oil and mushrooms to skillet. Sauté mushrooms about 5 minutes, or until golden brown. Add butter and garlic and sauté until butter is absorbed. In a small bowl, stir together lemon juice, soy sauce, and sugar. Add lemon juice, soy sauce, and sugar mixture to mushrooms, stirring until sauce is absorbed.

Snacks and Appetizers

► *Barbecue Chicken Wraps*
► *Tejano-Style Shrimp Cocktail*

Barbecue Chicken Wraps

Serves 4 | Preparation time: 45 minutes | Easy

Great texture (bacon, tortilla, and chicken), varied temperature, and spice (jalapeño peppers and barbecue sauce) provide all the necessities for stimulation of the normal sensory system of the mouth. This recipe was given to us by a patient with total loss of smell and inability to recognize any flavors.

INGREDIENTS

2 chicken breasts, cooked and shredded
2 cups barbecue sauce
¼ cup crumbled bacon
4 10-inch flour tortillas
1 cup shredded cheddar cheese
1 cup creamy deli coleslaw
½ cup chopped pickles
¼ cup chopped jalapeño peppers

PREPARATION

In a saucepan, simmer chicken and barbecue sauce together for about 10 minutes. Add bacon and stir until heated through. Remove from heat.

Heat tortillas as directed on package. Spoon chicken mixture into center of each tortilla. Top with ¼ of the cheese. Add a spoonful of coleslaw to each side of the tortilla, and add chopped pickles and jalapeños as desired. Fold up the bottom of the tortilla and roll it up. Serve immediately.

Tejano-Style Shrimp Cocktail

Serves 6 as a main course, 8 as an appetizer I Preparation time: 1 hour I Easy

The patient who submitted this recipe explained that it is one of the few that she and her husband enjoy together. She frequently has to prepare different foods for each of them, both because he tends to be fussy and because she has a smell and taste impairment.

INGREDIENTS

1 pound cooked medium shrimp, chilled
½ large cucumber, cut into ½-inch cubes
½ large tomato, cut into ½-inch cubes
1½ serrano peppers, halved lengthwise, deseeded and deveined, finely minced
1 bunch green onions, thinly sliced, including some of the green tops
¼ cup finely chopped, fresh cilantro
1 8-ounce can of tomato sauce
2 tablespoons white vinegar
1 lime

PREPARATION

Combine shrimp, cucumber, tomato, serrano peppers, onions, and cilantro in a large bowl. Stir in tomato sauce and vinegar. Squeeze lime over mixture. Serve in large bowl or in margarita or martini glasses.

Fish and Seafood

- ► *Pescado en Mojo de Ajo (Fish in Garlic Sauce)*
- ► *Spicy Grilled Shrimp*
- ► *Tandoori Salmon*

Pescado en Mojo de Ajo (Fish in Garlic Sauce)

Serves 4 | Preparation time: 30 minutes | Moderately challenging

This recipe, submitted by a patient, provides interesting texture, heat, and good basic taste, especially sour and tart from the lime.

INGREDIENTS
4 skinless fillets of any mild white fish
¼ cup flour
8 tablespoons clarified butter
4 cloves garlic, minced
Juice of 1 lime
4 lime wedges

PREPARATION
Dust fish fillets lightly with flour. Heat 2 teaspoons of the clarified butter in a frying pan until very hot but not smoking. Sauté the fish until lightly browned. Remove the fish from the pan, and add additional butter as desired (you will likely want about 2 to 3 tablespoons of melted butter per fillet to sauce the finished dish). Add garlic to the pan and sauté until it is light brown. Do not allow the garlic to burn, but do allow it to take on some color and become slightly crisp. Squeeze in the lime juice. Pour the hot butter, garlic, and lime mixture over the fish. Garnish with lime wedges, and serve.

Spicy Grilled Shrimp

Serves 6 | Preparation time: 45 minutes | Easy

This patient-submitted recipe is an ideal combination of great texture (the large shrimp), spice (cayenne pepper), and basic taste (coarse lime salt and lemon juice).

INGREDIENTS

1 large clove garlic
1 tablespoon coarse lime salt
½ teaspoon cayenne pepper
1 teaspoon paprika
2 tablespoons olive oil
2 teaspoons lemon juice
2 pounds large shrimp, peeled and deveined
8 lemon wedges for garnish

PREPARATION

Preheat grill to medium heat.

In a small bowl, crush the garlic with the lime salt. Mix in cayenne pepper and paprika. Next, stir in olive oil and lemon juice to form a paste. In a large bowl, toss the shrimp with the paste until evenly coated.

Lightly oil grill grate. Grill shrimp for 2 to 3 minutes per side, until opaque. Transfer to a serving dish, garnish with lemon wedges, and serve.

Tandoori Salmon

Serves 4 | Preparation time: 5 hours, including time to marinate |
Moderately challenging

This is one of our most popular tested recipes. One hundred percent of our taste testers enjoyed the original recipe. Those with normal smell and taste did not like the variations noted in the box, but 100 percent of those with impaired smell enjoyed the first variation and 50 percent enjoyed the second variation. This recipe has a great amount of all the recommended ingredients for those with smell and secondary taste impairment: texture, temperature, spice (mustard seeds, cumin seeds, cayenne pepper, jalapeño peppers), and basic tastes (salt, ginger).

INGREDIENTS
4 6-ounce salmon fillets, preferably wild Alaskan
2 teaspoons cayenne pepper
1 teaspoon salt
½ teaspoon freshly ground black pepper
2 teaspoons coriander seeds
2 teaspoons cumin seeds
2 teaspoons mustard seeds (black, yellow, or a combination)
½ cup plain yogurt
2 tablespoons chopped fresh ginger
2 cloves garlic, chopped
2 jalapeño peppers, seeded and chopped
Coarsely chopped cilantro for garnish

PREPARATION
Place salmon fillets in a shallow dish just large enough to fit all in a single layer. Combine cayenne pepper with salt and black pepper. Sprinkle mixture evenly over fish. Let stand 30 minutes.

Meanwhile, combine coriander, cumin, and mustard seeds in a small skillet over medium-high heat. Toast, shaking pan often, until seeds pop and start to color but not darken. Transfer seeds to blender. Add yogurt, ginger, garlic, and jalapeño and grind until smooth. Spread mixture over fish. Cover and refrigerate 4 hours.

Heat oven to 450°F. Line baking sheet with heavy aluminum foil. Brush most of marinade off salmon, leaving a thick glaze. Transfer fish to foil-lined baking sheet and roast until cooked to taste, about 10 to 12 minutes. The top should be almost crusty. If not, put fish under broiler quickly. Serve hot or warm with cilantro garnish.

Variations to Enhance Smell and Taste
TRY ADDING: ½ seeded, minced jalapeño pepper and ⅛ teaspoon cayenne pepper *or* 1 tablespoon ginger

Chicken

- ► *Lemon Pepper Grilled Chicken*
- ► *Tortilla Soup*

Lemon Pepper Grilled Chicken

Serves 5 | Preparation time 3½ hours, including time to marinate | Easy

This is another popular patient-submitted recipe. If you enjoy the taste of lemon with chicken, the addition of mustard, lemon pepper, and wine may prove to be a real hit, as it was with this patient and her family. Those with impaired smell and taste can add additional lemon pepper and mustard to their own portions to increase spiciness.

INGREDIENTS
¼ cup lemon pepper
1 tablespoon dry mustard
1 tablespoon dried rosemary
5 skinless, boneless chicken breast halves
4 cloves garlic, crushed
4 tablespoons fresh lemon juice
3 cups dry white wine

PREPARATION
Mix lemon pepper, dry mustard, and dried rosemary in a small bowl. Place chicken breast halves in a medium bowl. Rub with garlic. Add the lemon pepper mixture and rub into chicken. Pour in lemon juice and dry white wine. Cover and refrigerate at least 3 hours before grilling. Preheat outdoor grill for high heat and lightly oil the grates. Grill the marinated chicken breasts until meat is no longer pink and juices run clear, or to desired doneness.

Tortilla Soup

Serves 8 | Preparation time: 2 hours | Moderately challenging

This soup recipe, the only one in the book, was given to us by a patient. If you enjoy spicy soups, this is the recipe for you. It has great texture, varied temperature, spice, and some basic tastants—all the ingredients for those with smell and taste impairment. The amount of both spice and texture (tomatoes and chicken) can be varied, depending on your preference.

INGREDIENTS

6 tablespoons vegetable or olive oil
12 corn tortillas, cut in strips
8 cloves garlic, minced
1 medium red onion, chopped
½ cup chopped, fresh cilantro
28 ounces diced tomatoes
8 cups chicken stock
2½ tablespoons cumin
3 bay leaves
2 tablespoons chili powder
1½ teaspoons salt
1 teaspoon cayenne pepper
2 pounds cooked chicken breasts, cubed

Garnishes
8 ounces shredded Monterey Jack cheese
2 medium fresh avocados, cubed
3 corn tortillas, sliced thin and fried until crisp

PREPARATION

In a large nonstick pot, heat oil over medium high heat. Add the tortillas strips, garlic, onion, and cilantro to the pot and sauté for 3 to 5 minutes. Stir in the tomatoes. Bring to a simmer; add chicken stock, cumin, bay leaves, and chili powder. Bring to a boil. Reduce heat and add salt and cayenne pepper. Simmer for 45 to 60 minutes. Remove bay leaves and stir in the chicken. Garnish each bowl with cheese, avocado, and crispy tortillas just before serving.

Beef

- ▶ *Barbecued Ground Beef*
- ▶ *Enchilada Casserole*
- ▶ *Stuffed Green Peppers*
- ▶ *Teriyaki Onion Burgers*
- ▶ *Traditional Meatloaf*

Barbecued Ground Beef

Serves 6 | Preparation time: 1 hour | Easy

This recipe can be enjoyed by all. The texture is excellent, and the spices (mustard, ketchup, and vinegar) can be increased for those with more impaired smell and taste.

INGREDIENTS
1 pound ground beef
1 cup chopped green pepper
1 cup diced onion
1 cup diced carrot
1 cup diced celery
2 tablespoons prepared mustard
1 cup ketchup
1 tablespoon vinegar
2 tablespoon liquid smoke
1 teaspoon cloves
1 teaspoon salt

PREPARATION
Brown meat and mix in the rest of the ingredients. Simmer on low for 30 minutes until the vegetables are tender. Serve on toasted hamburger buns.

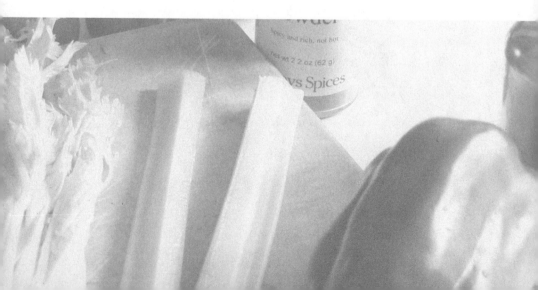

Enchilada Casserole

Serves 6 | Preparation time: 1½ hours | Challenging

This recipe was given to us by a patient of Hispanic descent who loves enchiladas. Many Mexican dishes are ideal for those with smell and taste impairment, because they often have ideal texture, temperature, and spice levels. Pepper, chili powder, and cumin can always be increased if the original recipe is not satisfactory. This is an excellent recipe for anyone who enjoys spicy food.

INGREDIENTS

Sauce
¼ cup vegetable or olive oil
2 tablespoons flour
3 cups hot water
2 tablespoons chili powder
2 teaspoons salt
1 teaspoon pepper
1 teaspoon garlic powder
1½ teaspoons cumin

Enchiladas
1 pound lean ground beef
1 large white onion, chopped
2 tablespoons chili powder
½ tablespoon garlic powder
½ teaspoon cumin
1 teaspoon salt
1 teaspoon pepper
12 corn tortillas
2 8-ounce packages of shredded cheddar cheese

PREPARATION

Preheat oven to 350°F. In a large skillet, heat 1 tablespoon oil. When oil is very hot (but not smoking), add the flour, stirring constantly until it is copper colored. When flour and oil mixture is heated through and very thick, add the hot water, stirring constantly. Next, add the chili powder and continue to stir constantly. Add salt, pepper, garlic powder, and cumin. Reduce heat to low and simmer about 10 minutes, stirring occasionally. Sauce will thicken as it cooks.

In another skillet, brown ground beef with onion, chili powder, garlic powder, cumin, and salt and pepper. Cook well and set aside.

In another small skillet, add the remainder of the vegetable or olive oil. Heat oil until very hot but not smoking. Add one tortilla, and lightly fry on one side. As soon as bubbles appear, turn the tortilla over and repeat. Remove each tortilla to drain on paper towels. Next, coat each tortilla evenly with the sauce mixture and place in a deep 13 x 9 inch baking dish. Cover bottom of baking dish with a layer of tortillas and add a layer of meat mixture. Sprinkle with a layer of cheese and repeat tortilla, sauce, meat, and cheese layers until the baking dish is full, ending with a final cheese layer on the top. Cover baking dish with aluminum foil and bake for 30 to 40 minutes, until cheese is melted and casserole is bubbling.

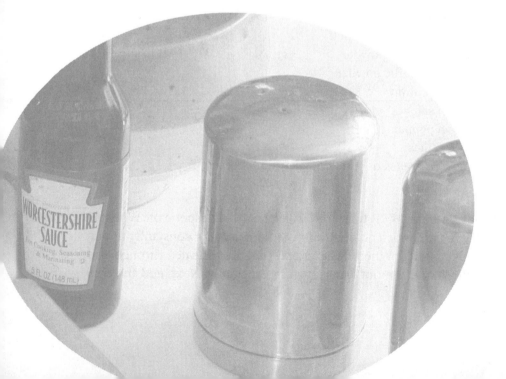

Stuffed Green Peppers

Serves 6 | Preparation time: 1½ hours | Moderately challenging

If you like peppers, the combination of good texture, spices (Worchester sauce, black pepper, and cumin), and basic taste (umami in the tomatoes and regular salt) in this recipe may be just what you are looking for. This recipe is also popular among people with normal smell and taste.

INGREDIENTS
6 large green bell peppers
1½ pounds ground beef
1 cup chopped onion
1 poblano pepper, chopped
1 16-ounce can diced tomatoes
1¼ cup water
1 teaspoon Worcestershire sauce
1½ teaspoons salt
1 teaspoon garlic powder
1½ teaspoon black pepper
1 teaspoon cumin
1 cup uncooked instant white rice
1 cup shredded cheddar cheese (or your personal favorite)

PREPARATION
Preheat oven to 350°F. Cut off the tops of the bell peppers and set aside to use later. Clean out the seeds and membranes in the pepper bottoms. In a skillet over medium high heat, cook the ground beef, onion, and poblano pepper until meat is done and vegetables are tender. Drain the grease from the beef mixture. Add tomatoes, 1 cup water, Worcestershire sauce, salt, garlic powder, black pepper, and cumin to the skillet, and bring to a boil. Add uncooked instant rice. Turn off heat. Add cheese to skillet, and stir well. Stuff the bell peppers with the beef, vegetable, and rice mixture and replace the pepper tops. Pour ¼ cup of water into a deep roasting pan. Set peppers in the roasting pan. Cover pan with aluminum foil and bake for 45 minutes.

Teriyaki Onion Burgers

Serves 4 | Preparation time: 30 minutes | Easy

This patient-recommended recipe has good texture and temperature qualities, but for some may require more normal basic tastes, such as sweetness and savory/umami than is provided in the recommended amount of teriyaki sauce. Those with smell and taste impairment might try adding sugar or MSG (such as Accent)—try adding a few "pinches," or up to ⅛ teaspoon, on your own portion.

INGREDIENTS
1 pound ground beef or turkey
¼ cup teriyaki sauce
1 3-ounce can French fried onions
4 slices cheddar cheese
4 split hamburger buns

PREPARATION
Preheat grill for high heat. Mix together beef, teriyaki sauce, and French fried onions in a medium bowl. Make 4 patties from the mixture. Lightly oil the grill, and grill the burgers 4 to 5 minutes on each side or until well done. Top with cheese and serve on buns.

Traditional Meatloaf

Serves 6 | Preparation time: 30 minutes, plus 1 hour and 15 minutes baking time | Easy

This recipe offers an excellent array of texture, temperature, and spices (vinegar, mustard, and Worcestershire sauce). It also includes lots of tomato and tomato paste, rich sources of the basic taste umami. If necessary, those with smell and taste impairment can add an additional pinch of MSG (such as Accent) to their own portions.

INGREDIENTS

1½ pounds ground beef
1 cup fresh bread crumbs
1 onion, finely chopped
1 egg, beaten
1½ teaspoons salt
¼ teaspoon pepper
½ can tomato sauce

Sauce
1 cup tomato sauce
1 6-ounce can tomato paste
½ cup water
3 tablespoons vinegar
2 tablespoons prepared mustard
2 tablespoons Worcestershire sauce
3 tablespoons brown sugar

PREPARATION

Mix together beef, breadcrumbs, onion, egg, salt, pepper and tomato sauce. Form into a loaf and place into a 7 x 10-inch loaf pan. Combine all sauce ingredients together and mix well. Pour sauce over the loaf. Bake at 350°F for 1 hour and 15 minutes.

Condiments

- ► *Bell Pepper and Dried Apricot Chutney*
- ► *Orange Balsamic Glaze*
- ► *Roasted Beet and Apple Relish*
- ► *Smoked Red Onion Vinaigrette*
- ► *Spicy Cranberry Relish*
- ► *Tropical Fruit Salsa*

All the condiments in this section were tested in our study, and we describe the level of enjoyment at the beginning of each recipe. We have given these recipes to many patients in our clinic and overall have received positive feedback on all of them.

Bell Pepper and Dried Apricot Chutney

Makes about 2½ cups chutney | Preparation time: 1½ hours plus at least 2 hours to chill | Easy

> Serve this chutney on lamb, beef, salmon, or chicken. The main recipe was enjoyed by 100 percent of our tasters with normal smell and taste function. One hundred percent of those with smell and tasted impairment enjoyed adding either additional curry powder or additional MSG (such as Accent), while 50 percent enjoyed the third variation.

INGREDIENTS

1 medium onion, chopped
1 red or orange bell pepper, cut into ½-inch pieces
1 cup dried quartered apricots
½ cup water
1 cup cider vinegar
½ cup plus 1 tablespoon sugar
1⅔ teaspoons curry powder, preferably Madras
½ teaspoon salt

PREPARATION

Bring all ingredients to a boil in a nonreactive 2-quart saucepan, stirring occasionally. Reduce heat and simmer, covered, until chutney is thickened but still saucy, about 50 minutes. Cool chutney, uncovered. Cover chutney and chill at least 2 hours and up to 1 week to allow flavors to develop. Stir occasionally.

Variations to Enhance Smell and Taste

TRY ADDING: 1 teaspoon curry powder *or* ¼ teaspoon MSG (such as Accent) *or* 2 tablespoons vinegar

Orange Balsamic Glaze

Makes 2¼ cups glaze | Preparation time: 45 minutes | Easy

A hit with those with smell and taste impairment, especially, due to the both the sweetness and tartness of the oranges. This glaze works very well with chicken and pork and can be made up to three days ahead of time and chilled.

In our study, 100 percent of those with normal smell and taste enjoyed the main recipe, and 75 percent enjoyed the first variation of additional orange preserves. None of those with normal smell and taste enjoyed the second and third variations, however. Interestingly, 75 percent of those with smell and taste impairment enjoyed the main recipe, but 100 percent enjoyed all of the variations.

INGREDIENTS
1½ tablespoons unsalted butter
1 cup finely chopped shallots
1 cup frozen orange juice concentrate, thawed
½ cup water
⅓ cup sweet orange preserves
⅓ cup balsamic vinegar
1½ tablespoons salt
½ tablespoons cracked black peppercorns
2 teaspoons finely grated orange zest

PREPARATION
Heat butter in a 3-quart saucepan over medium heat until foam subsides. Cook shallots, stirring until golden brown (about 5 minutes). Stir in remaining ingredients and simmer uncovered, stirring occasionally, until thickened and reduced to about 2¼ cups, about 25 minutes. Serve at room temperature.

Variations to Enhance Smell and Taste
TRY ADDING: 2 tablespoons orange preserves *or* 2 tablespoons balsamic vinegar *or* ¼ teaspoon MSG (such as Accent)

Roasted Beet and Apple Relish

Makes about 4 cups relish | Preparation time: about 3 hours, plus at least 2 hours additional time to chill | Moderately challenging

Lots of spice provided by black pepper and horseradish and the tartness of Granny Smith apples makes this relish an enjoyable experience for most who try it. One hundred percent of our tasters with normal smell and taste enjoyed the main recipe, but none of the variations. Seventy-five percent of those with smell and taste problems enjoyed the main recipe as well as added horseradish or MSG. Fifty percent enjoyed additional vinegar.

INGREDIENTS
3 medium beets (1 pound total with greens), trimmed, leaving 1 inch
    of stems attached
⅔ cup cider vinegar
2 tablespoons sugar
3 tablespoons salt
½ teaspoon black pepper
2 Granny Smith apples (about 1 pound total), cut into ¼-inch pieces
2½ tablespoons prepared horseradish

PREPARATION
Preheat oven to 425°F.

Tightly wrap beets in a double layer of aluminum foil and roast on a baking sheet in the middle of oven until very tender, 75 to 90 minutes. While beets are roasting, stir together vinegar, sugar, salt, and pepper in a large bowl until sugar and salt are dissolved. Add apples to dressing along with horseradish, and toss well. When beets are roasted, keep in foil package until cool enough to handle, about 20 minutes. Slip skins off beets and remove stems. Dice beets to ¼-inch pieces and stir into apple mixture. Cover relish and chill at least 2 hours and up to 3 days to allow flavors to develop. Stir occasionally.

Variations to Enhance Smell and Taste
TRY ADDING: ¼ teaspoon horseradish or ¼ teaspoon MSG (such as Accent) or 1 tablespoon vinegar

Smoked Red Onion Vinaigrette

Serves 8 | Preparation time: 2½ hours | Moderately challenging

This vinaigrette is very popular among those with both normal and impaired smell and taste. Those with smell and taste impairment often enjoy the two variations. Try it on salads and as a chicken marinade. It does require the use of a smoker for the onions.

INGREDIENTS

4 large red onions, sliced crosswise about ½-inch thick

¼ cup white vinegar

3 cups granulated sugar

¼ cup olive oil

1 tablespoon minced fresh thyme

1 teaspoon salt

½ teaspoon pepper

PREPARATION

Smoke red onions in a smoker on high heat for 1 hour, or purchase presmoked onions. In a tall, thick-bottomed stockpot, cover onions with white vinegar and sugar. Simmer for 1 hour, or until liquid is reduced by half. Cool completely. In a large blender, blend the onions with half of the liquid and drizzle in the olive oil, adding some of the reserved liquid if necessary to reach the desired consistency. Add thyme, salt, and pepper, and blend until well mixed.

> **Variations to Enhance Smell and Taste**
> TRY ADDING: ¼ cup vinegar or ½ cup sugar

Spicy Cranberry Relish

Makes about 2½ cups relish | Preparation time: 30 minutes, plus at least 2 hours to chill | Easy

This relish has a good amount of spicy serrano pepper and a tartness provided by lime juice and zest. For those with smell and taste impairment, it gives some excitement to the fish or chicken, which can be very bland to them by themselves.

INGREDIENTS

1 12-ounce bag (3 cups) fresh cranberries
1 teaspoon lime zest
2 tablespoons lime juice
1 medium red onion, chopped
½ cup sugar
1 teaspoon minced, fresh serrano pepper, including seeds

PREPARATION

In a food processor, pulse all ingredients until finely chopped. Cover relish; chill at least 2 hours and up to 1 week to allow flavors to develop. Stir occasionally.

Variations to Enhance Smell and Taste
TRY ADDING: 1 teaspoon serrano chili *or* ¼ cup sugar

Tropical Fruit Salsa

Makes about 2 cups salsa | Preparation time: 30 minutes | Easy

This salsa makes an excellent dip for tortilla chips. It is also a great topping for chicken, turkey, salmon, and ahi or yellowfin tuna.

INGREDIENTS

1 cup finely diced pineapple
½ cup finely diced firm, ripe mango
⅓ cup finely chopped white onion
1¼ teaspoon minced jalapeño pepper, including seeds
2 tablespoons fresh chopped cilantro
2 tablespoons fresh orange juice
2 tablespoons fresh lime juice
⅔ teaspoon salt

PREPARATION

Stir all ingredients together and refrigerate.

> *Variations to Enhance Smell and Taste*
> **TRY ADDING:** 1 tablespoon of orange juice and 1 tablespoon of lime juice *or* 2 teaspoons of minced jalapeño pepper *or* ¼ teaspoon MSG (such as Accent)

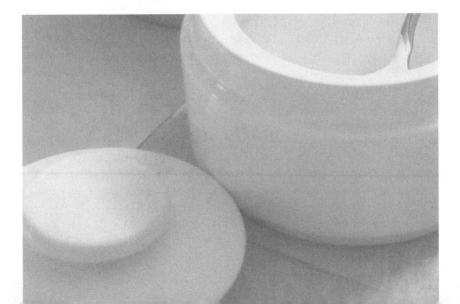

Marinades and Sauces

- ► Chicken and Beef Marinade
- ► Dr. Pepper Chicken Marinade
- ► Lemon Pepper Marinade for Chicken and Fish
- ► Spicy Steak Marinade
- ► Teriyaki Marinade for Beef
- ► Bourbon Barbecue Sauce
- ► Garlic Barbecue Sauce for Chicken, Beef, or Pork
- ► Honey Barbecue Sauce
- ► Spicy Barbecue Sauce

Introduction

Many of our patients have requested recipes for marinades and sauces because of their inexperience with food preparation. Using marinades is a simple way to enhance the flavor of fish, poultry, meat, and vegetables. The marinades in most cases emphasize spice and the basic taste of sweet, sour, and salty, which are usually normal in people with smell and taste disorders. Our food consultant chose the following marinades and sauces based on the inclusion of ingredients that have the ability to maximize the flavor of foods. We think everyone—whether you have a smell and taste impairment or not—will enjoy these recipes. Don't be afraid to modify them to enhance the flavors and tastes you enjoy the most.

Why and How to Use Marinades and Sauces

What's the secret to a perfect barbecue? Marinate, marinate, marinate. Un-marinated food is never as tender, juicy, or mouthwateringly delicious as food that has been soaked in a subtle or bold sauce before being seared over open coals. Although grilling gives you juicy, smoky meat, sometimes you want to add a little flavor to the mix. Do this with sauces and marinades, both of which add flavor and tenderness to anything you put them on.

Marinades are liquid and can be made out of pretty much anything. The most important ingredient is something acidic (such as lemon juice, vinegar, or yogurt) or fruity (particularly tropical fruit, such as papaya, pineapple, or kiwi). Both acids and the enzymes found in tropical fruit react with meat proteins to tenderize.

For minimal mess, use a resealable plastic bag; put all the ingredients inside, seal them up, and shake to combine.

For your safety, please follow these rules when using marinades:

► Always marinate food in the refrigerator, never at room temperature!
► Do not reuse marinades; if you want to make a sauce out of the leftovers, either boil them for at least 2 minutes, or make a separate batch for sauce.
► Brush off the extra marinade on your meat before putting it on the grill.
► If you're cooking with barbecue sauce, brush it on at the end of the cooking process so the meat can cook through without the sugars in the sauce burning.

Chicken and Beef Marinade

Makes 3½ cups | Preparation time: 10–15 minutes | Easy

| This marinade is an excellent flavor enhancement for chicken and beef.

INGREDIENTS
1 20-ounce bottle teriyaki sauce
1 12-ounce bottle of beer
¼ cup pineapple juice
Juice of 1 large lime
4 cloves garlic, minced
2 tablespoons brown sugar

PREPARATION
Mix all ingredients and pour over boneless chicken breasts or flank steak. Marinate at least 4 hours or overnight. Grill and serve. The finished product can also be frozen and reheated in the microwave.

Dr. Pepper Chicken Marinade

Makes about 4 cups marinade | Preparation time: 30 minutes | Easy

INGREDIENTS

1 can (14½ ounces) tomatoes
¼ cup finely chopped onion
2 teaspoons Worcestershire sauce
½ teaspoon allspice
¼ teaspoon salt
1 teaspoon freshly ground black pepper
½ teaspoon cayenne pepper
1 12-ounce can Dr. Pepper

PREPARATION

Puree tomatoes and add to a 1-quart saucepan with onion, Worcestershire sauce, allspice, salt, and peppers. Bring to a boil; simmer for 5 minutes, stirring occasionally. Remove from heat and stir in Dr. Pepper. Use to marinate chicken for at least 2 hours—overnight, if possible.

Lemon Pepper Marinade for Chicken and Fish

Makes ½ cup marinade | Preparation time: 15 minutes | Easy

INGREDIENTS
2 tablespoons olive oil
¼ cup fresh lemon juice
½ small onion, finely minced
1 clove garlic, minced
2 tablespoons chopped, fresh rosemary
Fresh, coarsely ground black pepper, to taste
Grated zest of 1 lemon

PREPARATION
Mix all the ingredients and use the marinade immediately with chicken or fish. Can also be used as a basting sauce, but bring to a rolling boil if using for basting after use as a marinade.

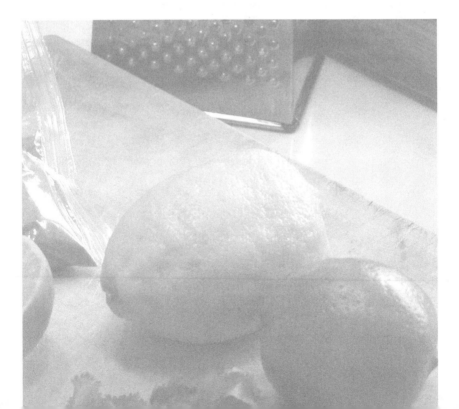

Spicy Steak Marinade

Makes 2½ cups marinade | Preparation time: 15 minutes | Easy

INGREDIENTS

12 ounces Guinness stout
4 ounces Jack Daniels whiskey
4 ounces peanut oil
2 ounces soy sauce
3 tablespoons Worcestershire sauce
1 tablespoon Tabasco sauce
2 cloves garlic, minced
1 teaspoon white pepper
1 tablespoon ground cinnamon
3 teaspoons salt
3 tablespoons honey

PREPARATION

Mix stout, whiskey, peanut oil, and soy, Worcestershire sauce, and Tabasco sauce in a saucepan. Bring mixture to a slow boil and add garlic, white pepper, cinnamon, salt, and honey.

Mix well before turning off heat. Allow to cool to room temperature. Use to marinate steak at least 2 hours and overnight if possible. If not using immediately, store in a glass jar in refrigerator for up to 1 week.

Teriyaki Marinade for Beef

Makes ¾ cup marinade | Preparation time: 10 minutes | Easy

INGREDIENTS

½ cup soy sauce
2 tablespoons Worcestershire sauce
1 tablespoon lemon juice
1 clove garlic, minced
2 tablespoons brown sugar
½ teaspoon ground ginger

PREPARATION

Combine all ingredients and mix well. Use immediately. Marinate steak at least 2 hours for more tender cuts of beef, and overnight for less tender cuts.

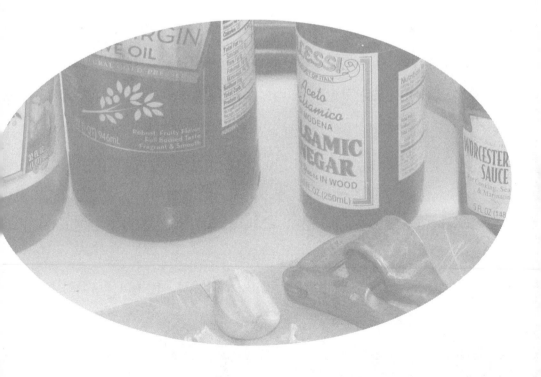

Bourbon Barbecue Sauce

Makes 2½ cups marinade | Preparation time: 1 hour and 15 minutes | Easy

> Use as barbecue sauce, or serve warm with grilled chicken or beef.

INGREDIENTS

3 tablespoons butter
3 tablespoons canola oil
1 cup chopped onion
½ cup bourbon
¾ cup ketchup
½ cup cider vinegar
½ cup orange juice
½ cup pure maple syrup
¼ cup dark unsulphured molasses
2 tablespoons Worcestershire sauce
½ teaspoon coarsely ground black pepper
½ teaspoon salt

PREPARATION

In a saucepan, melt the butter with the oil over medium heat. Add onions, and sauté until golden, about 5 minutes. Add remaining ingredients and stir to combine. Reduce heat to low and cook until thickened, about 30 to 45 minutes, stirring often.

Garlic Barbecue Sauce for Chicken, Beef, or Pork

Makes about 3½ cups sauce | Preparation time: 1 hour | Easy

INGREDIENTS
1 10¾-ounce can condensed tomato soup
1 8-ounce can tomato sauce
½ cup light molasses
½ cup vinegar
¼ cup vegetable oil
2 teaspoons Worcestershire sauce
2 tablespoons finely chopped onion
1 small clove garlic, minced
½ cup light brown sugar, packed
2 teaspoons seasoned salt
2 teaspoons dry mustard
2 teaspoons orange or lemon zest
1 teaspoon paprika
½ teaspoon pepper

PREPARATION
Mix all ingredients in a medium saucepan and bring to a boil. Reduce heat and simmer uncovered for 15 to 20 minutes. Brush on chicken or meat during last 15 minutes of grilling. Freeze extra sauce.

Honey Barbecue Sauce

Makes 3 cups sauce | Preparation time: 3½ hours | Easy

INGREDIENTS

1 cup dry white wine
3 tablespoons vinegar
2 tablespoons lemon juice
3 tablespoons Worcestershire sauce
¼ cup honey
2 cups ketchup
½ tablespoon Louisiana hot sauce
1 tablespoon liquid smoke
3 cups chopped onion
1 tablespoon chopped garlic
1 cup chopped sweet pepper
1 tablespoon salt
½ cup dried parsley

PREPARATION

Mix all ingredients in a large saucepan and bring to a boil. Simmer covered, over very low heat, for 2 to 3 hours.

Spicy Barbecue Sauce

Makes 3 cups sauce | Preparation time: 1 hour | Easy

Use as a basting sauce for grilled or baked ribs, pork chops, or chicken.

INGREDIENTS
2 cups water
¾ cup vinegar
¼ cup sugar
1 tablespoon Worcestershire sauce
¾ cup ketchup
1 cup finely chopped onion
1 teaspoon black pepper
1 teaspoon paprika
2 teaspoons salt
Dash of ground cayenne pepper or hot pepper sauce

PREPARATION
Mix all ingredients in saucepan and bring to a boil. Reduce heat and simmer for 30 minutes.

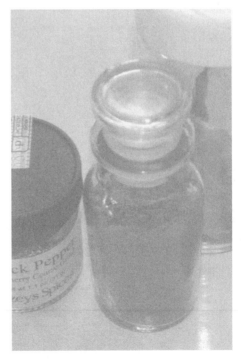

Tips for Holiday Meals

The holiday season is the time of year that we typically spend gathered with family and friends, often around meals. During the meal planning process, take into consideration the dietary needs of elderly guests and others—maybe even you—who may have an impaired sense of smell and taste. Remember to utilize the tips we have already presented emphasizing texture, spices, and presentation.

For example, if you are serving turkey, think about stuffing the cavity of the bird with onions, garlic, and herbs, or with apples, oranges, and apricots. Not only will this impart more flavor to the meat, but it will also ensure that the meat is very moist and tender. You can also enhance the flavor and taste of your turkey by stuffing garlic cloves and herbs under the skin prior to roasting. Also, try seasoning the skin of the bird well with coarsely ground pepper, sea or kosher salt, and garlic powder.

If you are preparing ham, consider a maple–brown sugar glaze and push whole cloves into the fat side of the ham before baking to enhance the aroma and flavor. You can also try adding roasted garlic or horseradish to mashed potatoes. Also, remember to include relishes, chutneys, and salsas that can be set on the dinner table for use as desired. Encourage your taste- and/or smell-impaired guests to try putting some condiments on their turkey, ham, or even mashed potatoes. Have a shaker of Accent handy since the MSG will enhance the existing flavors. Consider using the following recipes from this chapter as some of your holiday meal side dishes:

Bell Pepper and Dried Apricot Chutney (page 128)
Orange Balsamic Glaze (Great with turkey or ham) (page 129)
Roasted Beet and Apple Relish (page 130)
Spicy Cranberry Relish (page 132)
Tropical Fruit Salsa (page 133)
Tejano-Style Shrimp Cocktail (Elegant first course at any holiday meal) (page 107)
Horseradish Potatoes (Instead of plain mashed potatoes) (page 101)
Pickled Cucumbers and Onions (As a salad or appetizer course) (page 103)
Sautéed Mushrooms (As a side) (page 104)

All of these suggestions can be prepared as stated in the original recipes for your guests who have normal smell and taste. Set aside a portion or portions so that they can be enhanced as needed for any smell- or taste-impaired guests.

The sooner you begin this new culinary adventure with any family members with smell and taste impairment, the better you will know which flavors, textures, and presentations are appealing, and you will be better able to apply these preferences to all of your food preparation throughout the year.

Recipe Credits

Asian Chicken Salad recipe was originally published in *Gourmet/Bon Appétit* and is reprinted with permission. Copyright © Condé Nast Publications. All rights reserved.

Chicken Salad with Grapes and Walnuts recipe was originally published in *Gourmet/Bon Appétit* and is reprinted with permission. Copyright © Condé Nast Publications. All rights reserved.

Horseradish Potatoes recipe was submitted by Taste of Home's Fast Family Favorites and is reprinted with permission from *Allrecipes.com.*

Mushroom Medley with Ginger, Garlic, and Soy recipe was originally published in *Gourmet/Bon Appétit* and is reprinted with permission. Copyright © Condé Nast Publications. All rights reserved.

"Pickled" Cucumbers and Onions recipe is reprinted with permission from Brys Stephens, for *Cookthink.com.*

Tejano-Style Shrimp Cocktail recipe was submitted by Rey Garza and is reprinted with permission from *Allrecipes.com.*

Pescado en Mojo de Ajo (Fish in Garlic Sauce) recipe is reprinted with permission from *BakingShop.com.*

Spicy Grilled Shrimp recipe was submitted by SUBEAST and is reprinted with permission from *Allrecipes.com.*

Tandoori Salmon recipe is reprinted with permission from *www.spider kerala.com/kerala/recipes/ViewRecipe.aspx?RecipeId=327.* Please visit *www .spiderkerala.com/recipes* for more Kerala recipes.

Lemon Pepper Grilled Chicken recipe was submitted by BBQ BRIAN and is reprinted with permission from *Allrecipes.com.*

Barbecued Ground Beef recipe is reprinted with permission from *www.south ernfood.about.com/od/crockpotgroundbeef/r/bl59c.12.htm?p=1.* © 2009 by Diana Rattray, About, Inc. *www.about.com.* All rights reserved.

Stuffed Green Peppers recipe is reprinted with permission from *www.south ernfood.about.com/od/stuffedpepperrecipes/r/b130220q.htm.* © 2009 by Diana Rattray, About, Inc. *www.about.com.* All rights reserved.

Teriyaki Onion Burgers recipe was submitted by LUVMOORES and is reprinted with permission from *Allrecipes.com.*

Bell Pepper and Dried Apricot Chutney recipe was originally published in *Gourmet/Bon Appétit* and is reprinted with permission. Copyright © Condé Nast Publications. All rights reserved.

Appendix A

Smell and Taste Clinics

This appendix lists specialized smell and taste clinics and research centers that exist around the globe. There are eight known centers across the United States. Their websites are all satisfactory and provide good information about their qualifications, programming, and appointment scheduling.

United States Clinics

California
Chemosensory Perception Lab
University of California, San Diego
9500 Gilman Drive, Mail Code 0957
La Jolla, California 92093
Telephone: 858-622-5830
Website: *chemosensory.ucsd.edu/* (accessed January 22, 2010)

Nasal Dysfunction Clinic
UC San Diego Otolaryngology | Head & Neck Surgery
9350 Campus Point Drive
La Jolla, CA 92037
Telephone: 858-657-8590
619-543-3893 or 619-657-8594
Website: *health.ucsd.edu/specialties/surgery/otolaryngology/nasal/* (accessed January 22, 2010)

Colorado
Rocky Mountain Taste and Smell Center
University of Colorado Medical Center

4200 East 9th Avenue Box 205, UCHSC
Denver, Colorado 80262
Telephone: 303-315-6600
Website: *www.uchsc.edu/rmtsc* (accessed January 22, 2010)

Connecticut
Lawrence Savoy Taste and Smell Center
University of Connecticut Health Center
263 Farmington Avenue
Farmington, Connecticut 06030-3705
Telephone: 860-679-2459
E-mail: taste@cortex.uchc.edu
Website: *www.uchc.edu/uconntasteandsmell/* (accessed January 22, 2010)

Illinois
The Smell & Taste Treatment & Research Foundation
845 North Michigan Ave., Suite 990W
Chicago, IL 60611
Tel: 312-938-1047
Website: *www.smellandtaste.org* (accessed January 22, 2010)

Ohio
University of Cincinnati Taste and Smell Center
University of Cincinnati College of Medicine
222 Piedmont Avenue
Cincinnati, Ohio 45219
Telephone: 513-558-4152
Website: *www.ent.uc.edu/facilities/facilities.html* (accessed January 22, 2010)

North Carolina
Smell and Taste Clinic
Department of Psychiatry
Duke University Medical Center
201 Trent Drive
Durham, NC 27710
Web site: *www.medschool.duke.edu* (accessed January 22, 2010)

Pennsylvania

Monell Jefferson Taste and Smell Center
3500 Market Street
Philadelphia, Pennsylvania 19104
Telephone: 269-519-4700
Website: *www.monell.org* (accessed January 22, 2010)

University of Pennsylvania Smell and Taste Center
3400 Spruce Street
5 Ravdin Pavilion
Philadelphia, Pennsylvania 19104
Telephone: 215-662-6580
Website: *www.med.upenn.edu/stc* (accessed January 22, 2010)

Texas

Taste and Smell Disorders Clinic
1200 Lakeway Drive Suite 8
Austin, Texas 78734
Telephone: 512-261-7909
Website: *www.tastesmell.com* (accessed January 22, 2010)

Washington, DC

Taste and Smell Clinic
5125 MacArthur Boulevard NW Suite 20
Washington, DC 20016
Telephone: 202-364-4180
E-mail: *doc@tasteandsmell.com*
Website: *www.tasteandsmell.com* (accessed January 22, 2010)

Clinics Outside the United States

Australia

Center for Chemosensory Research
145 NIC Building
Australian Technology Park, Sydney
Australia 1430
Telephone: 61 2 9209 4083
Website: *http://www.chemosensory.com* (accessed January 22, 2010)

England

Royal National Throat, Nose, and Ear Hospital
330 Grays Inn Road
London, WC1X8A
Telephone: +44 (0) 207915 1300
Website: *http://www.royalfree.nhs.uk/index.aspx* (accessed January 22, 2010)

Germany

Dresden University Smell Dysfunction Clinic
74 Fetscherstrasse
Dresden, Germany D-01307
Telephone: +49 351 458 4189
Website: *www.tu-dresden.de/medkhno/hummel.htm* (accessed January 22, 2010)

Israel

The Institute for Nose and Sinus Therapy and Clinical Investigations
Wolfson Medical Center POB5
Holon, Israel 58100
Telephone: +972 3 5028618

Appendix B

Food Resources

This appendix lists some popular websites for information on and on-line purchase of spices and seasonings. This information was obtained from many of our patients and our food professional. Some of the seasonings and spices mentioned in the websites can also be purchased from your supermarket.

Global Palate (spices and blends)
Website: *www.globalpalate*.com (accessed January 22, 2010)

Leffingwell & Associates (extracts and spices)
Website: *www.leffingwell.com* (accessed January 22, 2010)

MSG Information
Website: *www.msginfo.com* (accessed January 22, 2010)

Nikken, Umami and Spices
BJ Harris Trading PPY Limited
Telephone: +61 2 9949 6655
Website: *www.bjharris.com.au* (accessed January 22, 2010)

Penzeys (seasonings and spices)
Brookfield, WI
Telephone: 800-741-7787
Website: *www.penzeys.com* (accessed January 22, 2010)

Serendipity (seasoning and spices)
Jess Hall Season Salt Company
P. O. Box 833
Weatherford, Texas 76086-0833
Telephone: 817-594-1617/800-460-7258
Website: *www.jesshall.com* (accessed January 22, 2010)

Spice Barn
Telephone: 866-670-9040
Website: *www.spicebarn.com* (accessed January 22, 2010)

(The) Spice House (spices, herbs, and seasonings)
Website: *www.thespicehouse.com* (accessed January 22, 2010)

Twang (flavored salt and spices)
San Antonio, Texas
Telephone: 800-950-8095
Website: *www.twang.com* (accessed January 22, 2010)

Victoria Gourmet (spices and blends)
Website: *www.worldpantry.com* (accessed January 22, 2010)
Telephone: 866-972-6879

Watkins (extracts, spices, and recipes)
Winona, Minnesota
Telephone: 507-457-3300
Website: *www.jrwatkins.com* (accessed January 22, 2010)

Appendix C

Recommended Reading

Aschenbrenner K, Hummel C, Teszmer, K, et al. The influence of olfactory loss on dietary behaviors. *Laryngoscope* 2008;118(1):135–144.

A very interesting and large study detailing the changes in dietary behavior such as appetite, eating out, making dinner, and attending parties in people with smell loss and altered taste. Individuals with a smell and taste disorder will identify with many of the people from the study.

DeVere R. Olfactory testing in the diagnosis of AD and other neurodegenerative disorders. *Practical Neurology* 2009;8(6)34–41.

This article discusses the value of smell testing in helping to make the diagnosis of mild cognitive impairment, Alzheimer's disease, Parkinson's disease, and Lewy body dementia. In addition, an abnormal smell test can also reveal important information about our ability to protect ourselves from environmental (smoke detection) and foodborne dangers.

Doty RL. Clinical studies of olfaction. *Chemical Senses* 2005;30 Supp 1:i207–i209.

This is a brief excellent summary article outlining the subject of causes of smell loss from an expert point of view.

Hawkes CH. Smell and taste complaints. *The Most Common Complaints Series*. London: Butterworth Heineman Publishers, 2002.

This is a very basic and readable book .It discusses all aspects of smell and taste symptoms and what tests and treatments are available.

Leopold D. Distortion of olfactory perception: diagnosis and treatment. *Chemical Senses* 2002;27(7):611–615.

This is an excellent article on the subject of bad odors (dysosmia) that occur in some smell disorders. It discusses the causes, outcome, and medical and surgical treatments of this unpleasant symptom.

London B, Nabet B, Fisher AR, et al. Predictors of prognosis in patients with olfactory disturbance . *Ann Neurol* 2008;63(2):159–166.

The article discusses the long-term outcomes of the common smell and secondary taste problems that a specialized clinic sees in everyday practice. This is the first study to obtain information over a period as long as 25 years. This study changed myths that most people with disorders of smell and taste do not recover.

Mattes RD, Cowart BJ. Dietary assessment of patients with chemosensory disorders. *Journal of the American Dietary Association* 1994;94(1): 50–56.

This articles discusses changes in food habits, nutritional intake, and body weight changes that occur in smell and taste disorders, and that negatively affect those with diabetes and hypertension.

Miwa T, Furukawa M, Tsukatani T, et al. Impact of olfactory impairment on quality of life and disability. *Archives of Otolaryngology Head and Neck Surgery* 2001;127(5):497–503.

This is an excellent article on how smell loss can impair a person's quality of life, health, and safety.

Schiffman S. Intensification of sensory properties of foods for the elderly. *Journal of Nutrition* 2000;130(4S Suppl):927S–930S.

This article discusses enhancing foods with various flavors and monosodium glutamate (MSG), which can improve food palatability and acceptance and reduce unpleasant taste symptoms in elderly people who are healthy or ill.

Appendix D

Internet Resources

This appendix provides a few Web sites for obtaining more information on smell and taste in general and on specific disorders.

MSG Information

Website: *www.msginfo.com* (accessed January 26, 2010)
This website provides easily understood information on MSG and has a list of frequently asked questions and basic answers on this subject.

National Institute on Deafness and Other Communication Disorders (NIDCD)

Website: *www.nidcd.nih.gov*
The smell and taste section of this website provides general information and is a source for research and research sites in the field.

Sense of Smell Institute

The Fragrance Foundation, Research and Education Division
Website: *www.senseofsmell.org* (accessed January 26, 2010)
This site provides good general information on smell and good articles written by important researchers and clinicians in the field.

About Neurologists

What is a Neurologist?

Neurologists are doctors with specialized training in disorders of the brain and nervous system, such as stroke, Alzheimer's disease, and multiple sclerosis. Almost all neurologic conditions can be treated, but few are curable or preventable. Most require highly skilled long-term management to maximize the quality of life for people with neurologic disorders.

A neurologist's training includes an undergraduate degree, four years of medical school, a one-year internship, and at least three years of specialized training. Many neurologists also have additional training in other areas—or subspecialties—of neurology such as stroke, epilepsy, neuromuscular disease, and movement disorders.

What Does a Neurologist Treat?

Common neurologic disorders include:

▶ Stroke
▶ Pain
▶ Headache
▶ Epilepsy
▶ Tremor
▶ Sleep disorders
▶ Alzheimer's disease
▶ Parkinson's disease
▶ Multiple sclerosis

▶ Brain and spinal cord injuries
▶ Brain tumors
▶ Amyotrophic lateral sclerosis (ALS, also called Lou Gehrig's Disease)

What Is the Role of a Neurologist?

Neurologists can provide principal care or consult with primary care physicians or other specialists. When a person has a neurologic disorder that requires frequent care, a neurologist is often the principal care provider. People with disorders such as Parkinson's disease, Alzheimer's disease, seizure disorders, or multiple sclerosis may use a neurologist as their principal care doctor.

In a consulting role, a neurologist will diagnose and treat a neurologic disorder and then advise the primary care doctor managing the person's overall health. For example, a neurologist may act in a consulting role for conditions such as stroke, concussion, or headache.

Neurologists can recommend surgical treatment, but they do not perform surgery. When treatment includes surgery, neurologists may monitor the patients and supervise their continuing treatment. Neurosurgeons are medical doctors who specialize in performing surgical treatments of the brain or nervous system.

Appendix F

About the American Academy of Neurology and the American Academy of Neurology Foundation

The American Academy of Neurology (AAN), established in 1948, is an international professional association of more than 22,000 neurologists and neuroscience professionals dedicated to promoting the highest quality patient-centered neurologic care. For more information about the American Academy of Neurology and resources for people with neurologic disorders, visit *www.aan.com*. To sign up for a free subscription to *Neurology Now*®, the AAN's bimonthly magazine for people with neurologic disorders, visit *www.neurologynow.com*.

The American Academy of Neurology Foundation raises money to support vital research into the prevention, treatment, and cure of brain disorders. The AAN Foundation is committed to improving patient care, quality of life, and public understanding of the brain and other neurologic disorders. For more information or to support research on brain disorders, visit *www.aan.com/go/foundation*.

Glossary

Each area of medicine has a set of commonly used terms that aren't necessarily commonly understood by people new to the field. The following are the major terms related to smell and taste that are found in the chapters of this book, along with a brief definition for your reference. The first time a term is used in the book, we have bolded it in the text and included the definition on that page. When you run into the term again, you may use this helpful glossary to refresh your understanding.

Acetylcholine One of a number of chemicals called neurotransmitters that relay signals in the brain and the junction between a nerve and muscle. Acetylcholine plays a role in a number of the body's physical responses, including stimulation of the salivary gland to release saliva. It also stimulates muscles to contract when we want them to move.

Alpha-synuclein A protein found in normal nerve cells. Its function remains unknown. It is abnormal and appears to be the source for smell loss when it accumulates in the olfactory bulb, tracts, and medial temporal lobe, which is the area of the brain that stores personal memories, general knowledge and facts, and recognizes odors. It is often found in people with Parkinson's disease and related disorders.

Alzheimer's disease The most common cause of dementia in people aged 65 and older; a progressive cognitive disorder that interferes with memory, insight, and judgment.

Aneurysm A weakened, bulging area in an artery. Some aneurysms put pressure on surrounding brain tissue. Others can rupture, flooding the brain with blood. Most aneurysms do not rupture, but those that do are life-threatening.

Aura An unusual sensation, sense of dread, or hallucination experienced by some people with seizure disorders before the seizure begins. This term is used to describe a phenomenon experienced by some people at the beginning of a migraine headache. The term visual or sensory aura is used when a person with migraine develops either flashing lights or numbness and tingling before a headache begins.

Axon A long, slender projection of a nerve cell that conducts electrical impulses, sending signals to and from the brain. Cilia project from one end of the olfactory receptor cells, collecting odor information, while axons project from the other, transmitting this information to the brain.

Bell's palsy A neurologic disorder that causes inflammation of the facial nerve (seventh cranial nerve). It causes partial or total paralysis of the facial muscles on one side of the face and alters basic taste (sweet, sour, bitter, salty, and umami) on the same side of the tongue as the facial paralysis.

Chorda tympani The nerve that joins the fifth nerve to the seventh nerve and carries basic taste information from the front two-thirds of the tongue.

Cilia Microscopic hairs found within the nasal smell organ (different from the larger nose hairs found near the opening of the nostril). These tiny hairs, bathed in the mucous of the nose, project from the olfactory receptor cells, capturing odors as they enter the nose and beginning the process of transmitting the odors to the brain.

Computed tomographic (CT) scanning A method of examining organs in the body by scanning them with x-rays and then using a computer to construct a series of three-dimensional cross-section images.

Congenital anosmia Complete absence of the sense of smell from birth.

Cranial nerves Twelve paired nerves (one for each side of the body) that emerge directly from the brainstem, primarily serving the motor and sensory systems of the head and neck.

Cribriform plate A bone in the front of the skull directly above the smell organ in the nose. It has many tiny holes through which the olfactory nerve fibers travel to reach the inside of the skull.

Dementia with Lewy bodies A progressive brain disorder showing early features of visual hallucinations and memory loss and later development of impaired judgment and reasoning. Features similar to Parkinson's disease, such as stiffness, slow movement, and tremor, develop between up to one year before to within one year of memory and cognitive decline.

Dysgeusia The perception of a usually unpleasant taste triggered by any normal taste or developing without a known trigger. The taste is commonly described as metallic in quality.

Dysosmia The perception of a smell, usually unpleasant, that may be triggered by a normal smell or arise without a known trigger.

Facial nerve (seventh cranial nerve) This nerve controls the muscles of facial expression and basic taste (sweet, sour, bitter salty, and umami) from the front two-thirds of the tongue by way of the chorda tympani nerve.

Foliate papillae Tiny bumps on the front and side edges of the tongue that contain taste buds. They are not easily seen by the naked eye.

Frontal lobe This structure makes up the front one-third of the brain. It is very important in our ability to reason, plan, judge, have insight, be attentive, behave appropriately, and recognize and identify everyday odors.

Fungiform papillae Small bumps on the center and front of the tongue that contain taste buds. They are not well seen with the naked eye.

Gastroesophageal reflux disease (GERD) A common medical condition caused by gastric acid spilling out of the stomach and traveling up the esophagus into the mouth and throat. GERD causes heartburn and can also cause a bad taste in the mouth. When left untreated, GERD can cause many other medical complications, including esophageal ulcers, chronic pulmonary disease, and Barrett's esophagus (a change in the lining of the esophagus that increases the risk of developing esophageal cancer).

Glossopharyngeal nerve (ninth cranial nerve) A nerve that carries basic taste information from the back of the tongue and throat. It is also responsible for secreting saliva, swallowing, and receiving sensory information (pain, temperature, and touch) from the back parts of the tongue and throat.

Limbic system A complex set of brain structures that includes the hypothalamus, the hippocampus, and the amygdala. The limbic system controls many basic functions of the body involving emotion and motivation, including experiencing pleasure.

Lingual nerve A branch of the trigeminal nerve that runs along the base of the tongue and carries taste, temperature, texture, and spiciness information from the front two-thirds of the tongue. The taste sensation nerve fibers enter the chorda tympani nerve, which is a branch of the facial (seventh cranial) nerve.

Magnetic resonance imaging (MRI) A medical imaging technique used to visualize the body's internal structure and function. It provides contrast between the different soft tissues of the body, using a powerful magnetic field rather than the radiation that is used in computed tomographic (CT) scans and x-rays.

Medial temporal lobe An area of the brain necessary in the storage of personal memories, general knowledge, facts, and odor recognition.

Microvilli Antenna-like structures that arise from all the taste receptors and are located in each taste bud. Microvilli contact the food molecules on the tongue so that their taste can be identified.

Mild cognitive impairment (MCI) A mild form of memory loss or other cognitive impairment that does not usually impair activities of daily living. The cause is unknown. MCI that predominantly involves memory impairment can lead to Alzheimer's disease in 65 percent of cases over a five-year period.

Monosodium glutamate (MSG) A sodium salt that, unlike regular salt, has a very savory taste similar to meat broth. It is representative of the newly accepted type of taste called **umami.** MSG is naturally present in many foods, such as tomatoes and beef. Twenty percent of the population cannot taste MSG due to a genetic defect. It is very safe and rarely causes nasal congestion, eye tearing, or migraine headaches. Much of the worry about using MSG is exaggerated. It has the same sodium content as regular salt but is available in a low-sodium form called Accent.

Mucous membrane Linings for many body cavities — such as the nostrils — that contain lubricants and secretions. The nasal mucous membranes allow odors to dissolve so that the olfactory receptors can detect them.

Multiple sclerosis (MS) A neurologic disorder of the brain and spinal cord of unknown cause. It usually affects individuals between 15 and 50 years of age. Symptoms, including visual loss, numbness or weakness of one or more limbs, and poor balance, usually come and go but can be progressive.

Nasal endoscopy A procedure in which a slender tube with a camera at the end is passed through the nostril to examine the nasal passages and sinuses.

Nasopharynx The connection between the nose and the region behind the tongue and upper throat. Food molecules in the mouth reach the olfactory organ in the nose through this pathway.

Neurotransmitter A chemical that relays information from one nerve cell to another.

Olfactory bulb Located in the base of the forebrain (the front part of the brain), the olfactory bulb is where the olfactory nerves from the smell organ in the nose terminate, and where olfactory tracts within the brain begin.

Olfactory cells Specialized nerve cells found within the smell organ. Olfactory cells have an outer nerve process that is capped with cilia that contacts the nasal mucous membrane and an axon that forms the olfactory nerve on the way to the olfactory bulb.

Olfactory cortex This term refers to parts of the brain that receive smell information. It includes a number of different brain structures, such as the deep inner side of the temporal lobe and the amygdala (a structure deep in the temporal lobe). The olfactory cortex is responsible for odor identification and intensity, not the ability to detect an odor.

Olfactory nerve A collection of axons from many olfactory cells that travel through the cribriform plate on their way to the olfactory bulb.

Olfactory receptors Nerve cells (neurons) in the nasal smell organ that are responsible for receiving and transmitting information about smell. They are the largest family in the human genome.

Olfactory system The nasal smell organ, olfactory bulb, tracts and olfactory cortex.

Olfactory tract A narrow tract of white nerve fibers that extends from the olfactory bulb into various parts of the brain.

Orbital frontal lobe The front part of the frontal lobe that sits directly above the orbit (eye socket) of the inside of the skull. This part of the brain allows us to appreciate and develop emotional connections to odors.

Parkinson's disease A movement disorder characterized by resting tremor of one or both arms and legs, rigidity (stiffness), slowing of movements, and problems with walking and balance.

Peripheral neuropathy Injury to the peripheral nerves (those farthest out from the center of the body) of the nervous system, usually affecting the hands and feet. Diabetes is one of the most common causes of peripheral neuropathy. In diabetic neuropathy, injury to the sensory nerves of the hands and feet (most often the feet) produces tingling, numbness, and pain.

Plaques Abnormal deposits of protein between nerve cells in the brain. These deposits are made up of a protein called beta-amyloid, and are characteristic of Alzheimer's disease. Plaques of a different kind occur in multiple sclerosis. These plaques are areas of inflammation and scarring due to damage of the covering of nerve fibers in the brain and spinal cord.

Polyps Abnormal growths of tissue projecting from a mucous membrane.

Prefrontal lobe The front part of the frontal lobe, the part of the forebrain involved in reasoning, decision making, and controlling emotions.

Rhinitis Irritation and inflammation of some areas of the lining of the nose, commonly described as a runny nose.

Schizophrenia A serious psychiatric disorder that causes disturbances in thinking, perception, and emotions.

Sjögren's syndrome A chronic autoimmune condition in which the white blood cells attack the glands that produce saliva. This condition affects as many as 4 million Americans.

Smell organ Located high up in the nasal cavity and made up of specialized nerve cells called olfactory cells. The main function of these cells is to identify odors and recognize different flavors.

Spinal fluid Also known as cerebrospinal fluid or CSF, this protective fluid circulates around the brain and spinal cord and acts like a cushion, protecting the spine and brain from injury and supplying nutrients to the brain.

Subfrontal region The bottom part of the frontal lobe closest to the bony base of the skull.

Tastants Substances that stimulate the sense of taste. There are five major tastants: sweet, sour, salty, bitter, and umami (savory).

Temporal lobe There are two temporal lobes, one on each side of the brain located at about the level of the ears. The temporal lobes allow for recognition of smells and sounds, as well as for meaningful and smooth speech and the retention of everyday memories.

Trigeminal nerve The name of the fifth cranial nerve. It carries information about touch, temperature, and pain to the brain from the face and inside the mouth, tongue, and teeth. It also carries information about texture, temperature, and spiciness of food.

Trigeminal nucleus The area in the brainstem where all sensory nerve fibers from the face and mouth end. All sensory information from the face, including touch, position, pain, and temperature, is carried to the trigeminal nucleus.

Trigeminal system The name given to the nerve system that includes the trigeminal nerve and its connections to the trigeminal nuclei in the brainstem, the thalamus, and the surface of the brain. This system provides information about pain, touch, and temperature of the face and inside of the mouth, and temperature, texture, and spice recognition of the food and drink we eat.

Umami A Japanese word meaning "tasty," umami is a relatively new term for one of the five basic tastes, roughly meaning "savory" or "meaty." (The other four basic tastes are sweet, sour, bitter, and salty.)

Vagus nerve (tenth cranial nerve) This nerve conveys sensory information about the state of the body's internal organs, such as the stomach, liver, and kidneys, to the brain. It also carries basic taste information from the back of the throat and larynx to the brain.

Index

Page numbers followed by *f* indicate a figure; numbers followed by *t* indicate a table.

Accidents, 64–65
Acetylcholine
  definition, 24
  and taste impairment, 24
Aging
  and smell disorder, 2–3
  and taste disorder, 22–23
Alcohol, and smell disorder, 11
Allergies, and smell disorder, 5–6
Alpha-synuclein, 14
Alzheimer's disease
  definition, 13
  in diagnosis and treatment, 50, 79
  and food preparation, 76
  and smell and taste disorder, xxi, 65–66
  and smell disorder, 2, 12–13
  and smell testing, 54, 78
American Academy of Neurology, xiii, 79, 165
American Academy of Neurology Foundation, 165
Aneurysm, definition, 50
Appetizers. *See* Snacks and appetizers
Asian chicken salad, 94
Aura, definition, 16
Axel, Dr. Richard, xxi, 34, 79
Axon
  definition, 34
  and smell system, 34

Barbecue chicken wraps, 106
Barbecued ground beef, 120

Beef
  barbecued ground beef, 120
  enchilada casserole, 121–122
  stuffed green peppers, 123
  teriyaki onion burgers, 124
  traditional meatloaf, 125
Bell pepper and dried apricot chutney, 128
Bell's palsy
  definition, 26
  and smell and taste disorder, 71
  and taste disorder, 26
Bourbon barbecue sauce, 142
Brief Smell Identification Test (B-SIT), 53, 54
B-SIT (Brief Smell Identification Test), 53, 54
Buck, Dr. Linda, xxi, 34, 79

Calcium, 77–78
Calvert, Marjorie, 81
Chemotherapy, and taste disorder, 24
Chicken
  lemon pepper grilled, 116
  tortilla soup, 117
Chicken and beef marinade, 137
Chicken salad with grapes, 95
Chorda tympani, definition, 26
Chronic liver disease, smell disorder and, 12
Cilia, definition, 5
Cirrhosis. *See* Chronic liver disease, smell disorder and

Cold-Eze, smell disorder and, 8
Computed tomographic (CT) scanning, definition of, 46
Condiments
    bell pepper and dried apricot chutney, 128
    orange balsamic glaze, 129
    roasted beet and apple relish, 130
    smoked red onion vinaigrette, 131
    spicy cranberry relish, 132
    tropical fruit salsa, 133
Congenital amosmia
    definition, 18
    and smell disorder, 18
Cranial nerves, definition, 21
Cribriform plate, definition, 3
CT (computed tomographic) scanning, defined, 46
Curried chicken salad, 96

Dementia with Lewy bodies, definition, 65
Dental procedures, taste disorder and, 32
Depression, 77
Diabetes
    and neuropathy, 12
    and smell and taste disorder, 69–70
    and smell disorder, 12
    and taste disorder, 30
Diagnosis and treatment
    by an ear, nose, and throat specialist, 49
    by a neurologist, 50
Doty, Dr. Richard, xx, 53
Dr. Pepper chicken marinade, 138
Dysosmia
    definition, 4,
    as life-threatening, 68
    and smell disorder, 7
Dysosmia, treatment for
    prescription medications, 67
    saline solution, 66–67

surgical removal of the smell organ in the nose, 67–68

Ear, nose, and throat (ENT) specialist
    diagnosis and treatment, 49
    examination, 50
Education
    about food preparation, 73–74
    about treatment, 62
Electrical testing
    and legal cases, 56
    olfactory evoked potentials (OEP) test, 55–56
Enchilada casserole, 121–122
ENT specialist. See Ear, nose, and throat (ENT) specialist
Examination
    by an ear, nose, and throat specialist, 50
    by a neurologist, 50

Facial nerve, defined, 51
FASEB (Federation of American Societies for Experimental Biology), 63
FDA. See U.S. Food and Drug Administration (FDA)
Federation of American Societies for Experimental Biology (FASEB), 63
Fish and seafood
    pescado en mojo de ajo (fish in garlic sauce), 110
    spicy grilled shrimp, 111
    tandoori salmon, 112–113
Fish in garlic sauce (pescado en mojo de ajo), 110
Foliate papillae
    definition, 40
    and taste system, 40–41
Food and spice combinations, 88t
Food preparation
    for altered taste, 76–77

and Alzheimer's disease, 76
combinations, foods and
    spices, 88*t*
education about, 73–74
enhancing taste, 74*t*
flavorings and extracts, 85–86
fruit preserves, 83
for moderate to severe smell
    loss, 76
and MSG, 75, 82
and Parkinson's disease, 76
for partial smell loss, 75–76
patient recommendations, 88
seasonings, 83
spices, 88
"tweaks," 82
umami compounds, 83-84, 87–88*t*
Food resources, 157–158
Frontal lobe, definition, 6
Fungiform papillae
    definition, 40
    and taste system, 40–41

Garlic barbecue sauce for chicken,
    beef, or pork, 143
Gastroesophageal reflux disease
    (GERD)
    definition, 30
    and smell and taste disorder, 70–71
    and taste disorder, 30
General anesthesia, and taste disor-
    der, 32
GERD. *See* Gastroesophageal reflux
    disease (GERD)
Glossopharyngeal nerve, defined, 51
Green chili ginger rice, 100

Holiday tips, 148–149
Honey barbecue sauce, 144
Hormones, 68–69
Horseradish potatoes, 101
Hypothyroidism, smell disorder
    and, 11

Injuries, head and nose, smell
    disorder and, 6–7
Internet resources, 161

Kidney function, smell disorder and, 12

Larynx surgery, taste disorder and, 32
Lemon pepper grilled chicken, 116
Lemon pepper marinade for chicken
    and fish, 139
Lewy body disease
    and dementia, 65
    and smell and taste disorder, xxi,
        65–66
    and smell disorder, 15
    and smell testing, 78
Limbic system
    definition, 37
    and memory, 37–38
    and smell system, 38
Linforth, Dr. Rob S. T., 43
Lingual nerve, definition, 32
Liver and kidney disorders, and taste
    disorder, 29

Magnetic resonance imaging (MRI)
    definition, 16
    and taste impairment, 28
    tumor in temporal lobe, 29*f*
Marinades and sauces
    bourbon barbecue sauce, 142
    chicken and beef marinade, 137
    Dr. Pepper chicken marinade, 138
    garlic barbecue sauce for chicken,
        beef, or pork, 143
    honey barbecue sauce, 144
    introduction to, 136
    lemon pepper marinade for
        chicken and fish, 139
    safety rules for, 136
    spicy barbecue sauce, 145
    spicy steak marinade, 140
    teriyaki marinade for beef, 141

MCI (mild cognitive impairment), 13
Medial temporal lobes, definition, 50
Medications
    change or reduction, 62–63
    and smell disorder, 7–10
    and taste disorder, 21–22, 25*t*
Memory, smell system and, 37
Microvilli
    definition, 40
    and taste system, 40
Migraine
    and smell disorder, 17
    and taste disorder, 28
Mild cognitive impairment (MCI), definition, 13
Monosodium glutamate (MSG)
    in cooking, 63–64
    definition, 63
    safety of, 75
    as salt replacement, 76
MRI. *See* Magnetic resonance imaging (MRI)
MSG. *See* Monosodium glutamate (MSG)
Mucus membrane
    definition, 34
    and smell system, 34
Multiple sclerosis
    definition, 15
    diagnosis and treatment, 50
    and smell and taste disorder, xxi
    and smell disorder, 15–16
    and smell testing, 78
    and taste disorder, 28
Mushroom medley with ginger, garlic, and soy, 102

Nasal endoscopy, definition, 50
Nasal polyps, 70
Nasopharynx, definition, 31
Neurologic disorders, and taste disorders, 26

Neurologists, 163–164
    diagnosis and treatment, 50
    examination, 50
Neurotransmitter
    definition, 24
    and taste impairment, 24
Nobel Prize, 2004, work on olfactory receptors, 34

Obstructive sleep apnea surgery, taste disorder and, 31
Odors, as cues to memory, 37
Odor training, 77
OEP (olfactory evoked potentials) test, 55–56
Olfactory bulb, defined, 4
Olfactory cells
    definition, 34
    and smell system, 34
Olfactory cortex, definition, 18
Olfactory evoked potentials (OEP) test, 55–56
Olfactory nerve, definition, 34
Olfactory nerve cells, 5*f*
Olfactory system, definition, 7
Olfactory tract
    definition, 35
    and smell system, 35
Orange balsamic glaze, 129
Orbital frontal lobe, definition, 11

Parkinson's disease
    definition, 14
    diagnosis and treatment, 50
    and food preparation, 76
    and smell and taste disorder, xxi, 65–66
    and smell disorder, 2, 13–14
    and smell testing, 55, 78
    and taste disorder, 22
Peripheral neuropathy, definition, 12
Pescado en mojo de ajo (fish in garlic sauce), 110

"Pickled" cucumbers and onions, 103
Pipette solution taste test, 57
Plaques, definition, 15
Polyps, definition, 46
Prefrontal lobe, definition, 11
Psychiatric disorders, and smell disorder, 17–18
Pungency, and taste sensation, 41–42

Q-SIT. *See* Quick Smell Identification Test
Quick Smell Identification Test (Q-SIT), 55

Radiation therapy, taste disorder and, 24, 26
Recipes
  beef, 119–125. *See also* Beef
  chicken, 115–117. *See also* Chicken
  condiments, 127–133. *See also* Condiments
  fish and seafood, 109–114. *See also* Fish and seafood
  holiday tips, 148–149
  marinades and sauces, 135–145. *See also* Marinades and sauces
  salads, 93–97. *See also* Salads
  sides, 99–104. *See also* Sides
  snacks and appetizers, 105–107. *See also* Snacks and appetizers
  taste surveys and, 82
  taste tests and, 82
Recommended reading, 159–160
Resources
  American Academy of Neurology, 165
  American Academy of Neurology Foundation, 165
  food, 157–158
  Internet, 161
  neurologists, 163

  recommended reading, 159–160
  smell and taste clinics, 153–156
Rhinitis, defined, 4
Roasted beet and apple relish, 130

Salads
  Asian chicken salad, 94
  chicken salad with grapes and walnuts, 95
  curried chicken salad, 96
  spicy Thai beef salad, 97
Saliva
  insufficiency, 71–72
  and taste system, 40
Sauces. *See* Marinades and sauces
Sautéed mushrooms, 104
Schizophrenia
  definition, 17
  and smell disorder, 18
Seafood. *See* Fish and seafood
Seizures
  and smell and taste disorder, 71
  and smell disorder, 16–17
  and taste disorder, 29*f*
Senses, ratings of importance, xix
Sides
  green chili ginger rice, 100
  horseradish potatoes, 101
  mushroom medley with ginger, garlic, and soy, 102
  "pickled" cucumbers and onions, 103
  sautéed mushrooms, 104
Sjögren's syndrome
  definition, 30
  and taste disorder, 30–31
Smell and Taste Center, University of Pennsylvania, xx
Smell and taste clinics
  coping strategies, 52
  international, 155–156
  treatment strategies, 52
  United States, 153–155

Smell and taste disorders
   and Alzheimer's disease, xxi, 78
   and depression, 77
   developments in the treatment of,
      xxi
   difficulties caused by, xix
   and food preparation. *See* Food
      preparation
   incidence of, xx
   and Lewy body disease, xxi, 78
   long-term follow-up studies, xxi
   and multiple sclerosis, xxi, 78
   and Parkinson's disease, xxi, 78
   safety tips, 72–71*t*
   and studies of, 44, 46
   symptoms of, xix–xx, xxi
   treatment. *See* Treatment, smell
      and taste disorder
Smell and taste, history of, 45–47
Smell disorder
   aging, 2–3
   alcohol, 11
   Alzheimer's disease, 2, 12–13
   causes, 2*t*
   chronic liver disease, 12
   congenital anosmia, 18
   diabetes, 12
   disorders of the nasal passages
      and sinuses, 3–6
   hypothyroidism, 11
   and injuries, head and nose, 6–7
   kidney function, 12
   Lewy body disease, 14–15
   medical disorders, 11–12
   migraine, 17
   mild cognitive impairment, 13
   multiple sclerosis, 15–16
   neurologic disorders, 12–17
   Parkinson's disease, 2, 14
   psychiatric disorders, 17–18
   seizures, 16–17
   smoking, 10
   toxins, 10

Smell organ
   and connections to olfactory bulb
      and brain, 35*f*
   definition, 34–35
   and food, 35
   and nasal cavity, 36*f*
   surgical removal of, 67–68
Smell or Odor Threshold Test, 55
Smell system
   axon, 32
   and limbic system, 36
   and mouth, 37
   mechanics of, 36–37
   and memories, 36
   mucus membrane, 32
   olfactory cells, 32
   olfactory nerve, 32
   olfactory tract, 33
   process, 31–36
   sniffing, 36–37
Smell testing
   and age, 53–54
   and Alzheimer's disease, 54, 78
   Brief Smell Identification Test (B-
      SIT), 53, 54
   and dementia with Lewy
      bodies, 78
   electrical testing, 55–56
   and multiple sclerosis, 78
   and Parkinson's disease, 55, 78
   Quick Smell Identification Test
      (Q-SIT), 55
   Smell or Odor Threshold Test, 55
   Sniffin' Sticks, 55
   summary, 57–59*t*
   University of Pennsylvania Smell
      Identification Test (UPSIT),
      53, 54*f*
Smoked red onion vinaigrette, 131
Smoking
   and cessation, 65, 69
   and smell disorder, 10
   and taste disorder, 26

Snacks and appetizers
    barbecue chicken wraps, 106
    Tejano style shrimp cocktail, 106
Sniffin' Sticks, 55
Sodium citrate buffer, 78
Spicy barbecue sauce, 145
Spicy cranberry relish, 132
Spicy grilled shrimp, 111
Spicy steak marinade, 140
Spicy Thai beef salad, 97
Spinal fluid, definition, 46
Stuffed green peppers, 123
Subfrontal region, defined, 46
Surgery, ear, nose, or throat, taste
        disorder and, 31–32

Tandoori salmon, 112–113
Tastants, taste sensations and, 43
Taste bud, 41*f*
Taste disorders
    aging, 22–23
    Bell's palsy, 26–27
    causes, 22–23
    chemotherapy, 24
    dental procedures, 32
    diabetes, 30
    gastroesophageal reflux disease, 30
    general anesthesia, 32
    larynx surgery, 32
    liver and kidney disorders, 29
    medical terms, 22*t*
    medications, 23–24, 25*t*
    migraine, 28
    multiple sclerosis, 28
    neurologic disorders, 26
    obstructive sleep apnea sur-
        gery, 31
    Parkinson's disease, 22
    radiation therapy, 24, 26
    Sjögren's syndrome, 30–31
    smoking, 26
    surgery, ear, nose, or throat,
        31–32

thyroid function, 28
tonsil surgery, 31
Tastes, basic
    bitter, 87
    salty, 87
    sour, 87
    sweet, 86
    umami, 87
Taste sensations
    pungency, 41–42
    studies of, 41–42
    tastants, 43
    temperature, 42–43
Taste Strips, 57
Taste system, 27*f*
    foliate papillae, 39
    function of, 39–41
    fungiform papillae, 39
    microvilli, 38
    saliva, 40
    taste bud, 41*f*
    tongue, 39, 39*f*
    trigeminal nerve, 39
    trigeminal nucleus, 39
    trigeminal system, 39
Taste testing
    pipette solution, 59
    summary, 57–59*t*
    Taste Strips, 59
    whole mouth taste test, 59*t*
Taylor, Dr. Andrew J., 43
Tejano style shrimp cocktail, 106
Temperature, and taste sensation,
        42–43
Temporal lobe
    definition, 6
    tumor in, 29*f*
Teriyaki marinade for beef, 141
Teriyaki onion burgers, 124
Thyroid function, and taste
        disorder, 28
Tongue, and taste system, 39, 42*f*
Tonsil surgery, and taste disorder, 31

Tortilla soup, 117
Toxins, and smell disorder, 10
Traditional meatloaf, 125
Treatments, smell and taste disorder
    accidents, 64–65
    Alzheimer's disease, 65–66
    for Bell's palsy, 71
    dementia with Lewy bodies, 65–66
    in diabetes, 69–70
    dysosmia. *See* Dysosmia, treat-
        ment for
    education, 62
    in gastroesophageal reflux dis-
        ease, 70–71
    hormones, 68–69
    medications, change or reduction,
        62–63
    for nasal polyps, 70
    Parkinson's disease, 65–66
    potential new, 77–78
    for saliva insufficiency, 71–72
    for seizure disorder, 71
    smoking cessation, 65, 69
    viral infections, 64
    vitamins, 68–69
Trigeminal nerve, *9f*
    definition, 8, 39
    and taste system, 37
Trigeminal nucleus
    definition, 39

and taste system, 39
Trigeminal system
    definition, 39
    and taste system, 38–39
Tropical fruit salsa, 133

Umami
    definition, 23
    compounds in cooking, 83–84,
        84–85*t*
University of Pennsylvania Smell
    Identification Test (UPSIT), 53,
    54*f,* 63
UPSIT. *See* University of Pennsylva-
    nia Smell Identification Test
    (UPSIT)
U.S. Food and Drug Administration
    (FDA), 9

Vagus nerve, definition, 51
Viral infections, 64
Vitamins, 68–69

Whole mouth taste test, 59t

Zicam
    and class-action lawsuit, 9
    and smell disorder, 8
Zinc glugonate gel, smell disorder
    and, 8

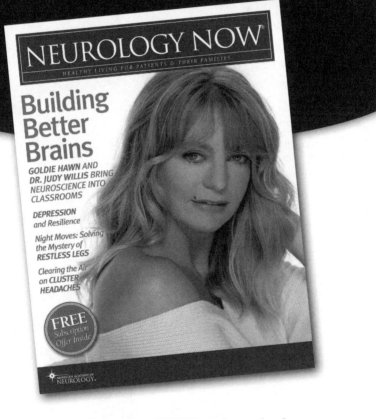
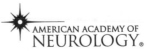